ENDING

VIOLENCE

QUICKLY

WARNING

Some of the techniques and drills depicted in this book are extremely dangerous. It is not the intent of the author, publisher, or distributors of this book to encourage readers to attempt any of these techniques or drills without proper professional supervision and training. Attempting to do so can result in severe injury or death. Do not attempt any of these techniques or drills without the supervision of a certified instructor.

The author, publisher, and distributors of this book disclaim any liability from any damage or injuries of any type that a reader or user of information contained in this book may encounter from the use of said information. This book is presented *for academic study only.*

Marc "Animal" MacYoung

A PROFESSIONAL'S GUIDE TO

ENDING

VIOLENCE

QUICKLY

How Bouncers, Bodyguards, and Other Security Professionals Handle Ugly Situations

Paladin Press • Boulder, Colorado

Also by Marc "Animal" MacYoung:
Cheap Shots, Ambushes, and Other Lessons
Down but Not Out (video)
Knives, Knife Fighting, and Related Hassles
Safe in the City (with Chris Pfouts)
Safe in the Street (video)
Street E&E
Surviving a Street Knife Fight (video)
Taking It to the Street
Violence, Blunders, and Fractured Jaws

A Professional's Guide to Ending Violence Quickly:
How Bouncers, Bodyguards, and Other Security Professionals
  Handle Ugly Situations
by Marc "Animal" MacYoung

Copyright © 1996 by Marc "Animal" MacYoung

ISBN 13: 978-0-87364-899-8
Printed in the United States of America

Published by Paladin Press, a division of
Paladin Enterprises, Inc.
Gunbarrel Tech Center
7077 Winchester Circle
Boulder, Colorado 80301 USA, +1.303.443.7250

Direct inquiries and/or orders to the above address.

PALADIN, PALADIN PRESS, and the "horse head" design
are trademarks belonging to Paladin Enterprises and
registered in United States Patent and Trademark Office.

Illustrations by Marc MacYoung

Visit our website at www.paladin-press.com

Contents

Introduction

"You are not a superman."

—Murphy's Law of Combat #1

was talking to a guy at my table at the Soldier of Fortune convention when the look on his face caused me to do a mental rewind about what I had just said. "Whoops, something's up here. Whaddi say?" We were talking about different self-defense courses that I recommend and why I thought they were good. Okay, nothing wrong there. What's with his expression then? He had this look of disbelief and amazement, mixed in with what can only be called a glimmering of hope. I stopped and looked at him expectantly.

"*You* were afraid?" he asked in shocked tones.

It didn't matter that I was standing in the middle of testosterone central. It didn't matter that I'm supposed to be some sort of street fighting expert. None of that really even came close to entering my mind. All I had to do was remember what it was really like out there, what it was like to have somebody actually try to kill me. It's a whole different ball game when the other side shoots back, and now and then the SOB is rude enough to get off the first shot too!

I looked at the guy and told him the stone cold truth.

"Man, I was terrified. The only time I wasn't scared was when I was either drunk or furious."

I thought about it for a second before muttering to myself, "That probably explains why I spent most of my time either drunk or furious."

Aw well, that's part of what being Animal was about. That and doing my damnedest to get laid a lot. With a shrug I looked back at him.

I watched this guy go through a metamorphosis in front of me. Hey, if someone *as big and bad as Animal* could say that he was scared, then it was okay to be scared. That's what the glimmer of hope was. Here was a guy who was trying desperately not to be scared by something that only sadists, psychos, and the *reeeaaallly* ignorant aren't scared of.

I watched this guy literally bloom in front of me as a whole mental domino process fell into place. Now he could learn how to take care of himself without feeling bad about feeling scared. Man, the dude was on his way.

I walked away from that conversation with two realizations. One is that despite my best efforts to convince people to the contrary, there are some people who believe that I'm some sort of fearless superman who regularly knocks bullets out of the air with my dick. If I ever find the guy who started that foul rumor, I'm going to strangle him, as such a thing flies directly into the face of Murphy's Laws of Combat #3 (Don't look conspicuous—it draws fire) and #10 (Try to look unimportant, because the bad guys may be low on ammo). Laws I heartily agree with.

Maybe I have knocked a bullet askew with that appendage, but I assure you it was not planned. In fact it was usually sort of a last-ditch effort to get off the line of attack. My most amazing feats have been directly related to the fact that the situation had gotten seriously ugly and it was my last option before being hospitalized—not, as some would believe, because I was a superman. (See Law #1 in Appendix G.)

I know better. I was there at the time.

It wasn't until later, though, that the second realization began to seep into my consciousness. It sort of built on top of the first, wormed its way through my subconscious, and eventually sidled up to the bar inside my brain and quietly ordered a beer. When I looked over at it, I suddenly realized what it was that had always set me apart from others when it came to violence. Ready? Here it is:

One way or the other, I wanted to end it as soon as possible . . .

That's it, folks. It doesn't matter if I was trying to kick ass or haul it, I wanted it over *now!* It doesn't take a rocket scientist to figure out that when someone is *trying* to hurt you, he might just succeed! And the longer you hang around under those sort of conditions, the more likely the chump is going to get lucky. By dropping that guy as fast as I could, I lessened the chances that he would get a piece out of me. Even when I had gotten to the point of where I was doing it professionally, I still maintained that mind-set.

Him. Down. Now. Game over.

Think about this for a moment, as it is one of the major differences between what is taught as martial arts and the reality of self-defense.

How much of what you have been taught flies directly into the face of this pearl of wisdom? Think about sparring. Is anyone really trying to end it? Or are they actually dancing around throwing punches, and the person with the most points at the end wins.

So does sparring teach you how to end a fight as quickly as possible? Not only no, but hell no. In fact, it teaches you to prolong it, to work your way up into a fight. *"Yeah, let me get two or three punches in and then I'll be warmed up and ready to go to town."*

Child, you try that against a street fighter and you're dog meat. (By the way, this is one of the reasons why I don't spar much, nor do I encourage my students to do so. It teaches the wrong thing. I believe in practicing, but not sparring.) The majority of all the fights I've seen between experienced fighters entail one guy getting an immediate advantage and exploiting it, whether that's pounding the bejeezus out of the dude or ramming the knife in again and again or repeatedly pulling the trigger. Once they start, they don't stop. *The object of the exercise is to make sure the other guy doesn't have a chance to strike back.*

When I would go ballistic all over some 6'8" dude, it wasn't because I was a kung fu superhero. It was simply because I knew that *the longer I stayed there under those circumstances, the more likely I was to get hurt.* If I didn't drop him immediately, he was gonna swat me like a bug. Every second that it went on increased my chances of getting hurt incrementally. If the chump happened to bring a weapon along, the chances of my getting hurt began to have those little numbers behind them that indicate to the X power.

Wrong! That is why I'd crawl all over the guy. Only by ending it immediately was I likely to come out of it unscathed. Once that switch was thrown and I was slamming and jamming, there was nothing fair, honorable, or civilized in what I did. Later, when violence had become part of my profession, while I wasn't out to maim my opponent anymore, I was still going to end the confrontation immediately and put him in a position where he couldn't hurt me.

See, I know something that most studly manly man martial artists and aggressive young bucks don't know. Quantum physicists talk about strong force, weak force, gravity, and magnetism as the four forces that run the cosmos. Well I happen to know that Murphy's Law is the fifth force of the universe. And anyone who has ever been out in the field knows that Murphy is real and he's waiting for you. *If it can go wrong, it will go wrong!* Maybe not always, but sooner or later we all get our turn in the barrel. If you haven't prepared for it, guess who's going for a little ride?

Your best chance of preventing Murphy's Law from nailing you is to get out of the danger zone as soon as possible. If you want to make a simile about it, try this: the less time you spend on the wrong end of a gun, the less chance you have of getting shot! The reverse is also grotesquely valid—the longer a violent situation goes on, the longer you're in front of the barrel, and all it takes is a little pressure in the right place. Remember, no matter how good you are, you can still be hurt.

A point that most would-be self-defense instructors miss is, not only does Murphy's Law work in spades in this business, but unlike in the martial arts school, when you're in a real situation, *the guy ain't on your side, bucko!* That's right, not only is he actively trying to hurt you, but he ain't gonna cooperate as you try to chuck him onto his head, karate punch him, or take your carefully designed shooting stance. In fact, don't be surprised when he actively does everything in his power to bring the almighty Murphy into your life! That's right—not only will he try to clobber you, but he'll try to mess up your attempts to do the same to him. Under these conditions, is it any wonder that our friend Murphy would show up? You bet he will! And sometimes in the nastiest way possible! (When did Murphy put that knife in the guy's pocket?! Ooops!)[1]

Maybe it was because I was ten years old the first time my switchblade malfunctioned, thereby leaving me in a bit of a bind, but I knew at a very early age that when it comes to violence, things go wrong, both due to simple Murphyisms and the other guy having a slightly different agenda than you.

Introduction

The object of the exercise is to get out of Murphy's reach as soon as possible. Pulling the trigger once in Russian Roulette is bad enough without hanging around for four more tries. When it came to violence, as far as I was concerned the only trigger that was going to get pulled was mine. And once I was done, the guy wouldn't be in any shape to pull anything else.

Consequently, I always planned my violence for both the shortest time possible as well as the simplest, most bulletproof moves I could find. When I streamlined it down to the bare basics, all I was doing was keeping it so simple that things were less likely to go wrong. I didn't rely on techniques, I relied on basic laws, like "gravity works." You can mess up a technique, but it'll take a long days walk before you can find an easy way to mess up gravity. I call that pretty bulletproof.

It is amazing to me that people are shocked when I say a fight should be over in three moves. They look at me like I've just asked them to jump up into a flying airplane or some other impossible task. I can't tell you how many times I've heard, "Well maybe for you, but you're a trained fighter." Nononononono! This is not a Kevlar-covered dick thing. It's just common sense!

Look at it this way. If he's lying on the ground clutching the root of all his fantasies, how much of a threat is he going to be to you? How about if he finds himself in a position where if he struggles he's going to get a broken arm (and that's before you really hurt him) or have a high-speed encounter with Mother Earth? Ah ha! A guy in any of these positions ain't much of a threat. If he continues to be a moron instead of cooperating, well, he chose Door Number 2. Got it?

Face it, if you are as big of a coward as I am, you will begin to see the sense of ending violent situations as quickly as possible. After all, a guy could get hurt doing this stuff! This is especially true if you do what I did and put yourself into a profession or regularly find yourself in situations where people are prone to try and off you. Such lines of work include bouncer, bounty hunter, bodyguard, hospital orderly (emergency room, psych ward, rehab, detox), correctional officer, halfway house monitor, security (in-house, contractual, store), military police, and law enforcement.[2] The quicker it's over, the less likely you are to get hurt. And that's what this book is about. You're going to learn the short-hand techniques that kept my skinny little ass alive out there against superior numbers, sizes, and firepower for so long. So get ready to change your thinking, buckaroos, 'cause it's reality check time!

By the way, before we go on, chant the mantra we all know so well by now about all my books . . .

Animal doesn't know everything. I gotta experiment with this.

You have to try things out yourself and find what works. If something in this book doesn't work for you, drop it faster than an annoyed tarantula and find what does!

Standard stuff by now, but I gotta say it or God knows how that little shmuck who's been trying to give me a big red "S" reputation will say. Like I said, if I ever catch that SOB . . .

ENDNOTES

1. The answer to that question is that Murphy put the knife there the second you didn't drop the guy fast enough to prevent him from getting it out.

2. For those of you who noticed the contradiction of being both a self-professed coward and a professional trouble hunter . . . where is it written that I have to be either consistent or smart?

CHAPTER 1

Escalato and Why You Shouldn't Play

"The conviction of the justification of using even the most brutal weapons is always dependent on the presence of a fanatical belief in the necessity of victory."
—Adolf Hitler

My brother Tim gave me a very good bit of advice about seven card stud: "If you don't have something good going by the fourth card, fold." The reason I share this information with you is to show you how a simple rule of thumb can save you loads of money. Try that strategy next time you play poker and see how much longer your money will last.

That attitude, by the way, flies directly in the face of how most amateurs play poker. It's also why they're called amateurs. They want to hang around to the very last, hoping that the magic straight flush fairy will come by and, *poof*, they're suddenly the winner. Yeah, right.

The reason I bring up the concept of poker is because the way that most people handle violence is damn near an

---

exact reenactment of an amateur poker game, especially the upping the stakes part. It's dumb enough in a poker game, but it's potentially lethal with violence.

Have you ever seen two poker players involved in an escalating round of betting? Instead of just plopping their money down and saying "call" and getting down to the business of who's going to come out on top, they "see and raise" it back and forth. Off they go into the wild blue yonder!

Now I can understand it when both guys are sitting there with good hands. What shocks me is how often this is played out when neither of them has a hand that is worth a bucket of piss. I have seen guys sit there with absolute garbage trying to convince the other guy to back down by raising the stakes. *What they were betting on was the other dude backing down before the stakes got too high, not the strength of their hands!*

Dumb move.

Many of these episodes come about because both of the guys feel they have so much invested in the pot that they can't pull out. This is especially true when booze is around to eat away at their common sense. Ohhh, Catch 22 here. Neither of them wants to show their hand for fear of losing, so instead they keep on raising the stakes. (It's like pushing down the gas pedal because you're afraid of going fast. Sheesh!) I have seen major money exchange hands over a pair of fives because of this very thing (the loser had a pair of threes, if you can believe it).

This is no longer poker; they're now playing "escalato." It's the feeling of having to "win" the hand and/or an overly developed sense of "investment" (read: because you can't back down) that leads to an upward spiraling game of escalato.

When it comes to violence, you do not want to become involved with this kind of game!

Most amateur violence comes about because of this stupid game of escalato. People have no clear-cut idea of what winning means, but by God they know they gotta do it. Think about how many times you've seen things escalate way out of control. This simple pattern is behind nearly 90 percent of all conflicts you'll encounter. Everything from a 3-year-old throwing a hissy fit to 90-year-old grandmothers having attitudes with one another. People get "locked in" and begin raising the stakes. Each round is more intense. It's a basic human pattern, no matter where you go.

In an escalating situation, what you've got is two people playing chicken by racing their cars toward the cliff. Each is hoping the other will jump out first so he/she can claim to have won. In case you haven't figured it out, betting your dick on the other guy doing the smart thing ain't a smart thing! The fact that both of them are there in the first place shows you how likely someone "doing the smart thing" won't happen! The really bad news is, if someone doesn't call a halt to it at some point, it's going to progress to the next step, which is violence.

Escalato is the most dangerous game in the world. In fact every year in the United States alone, more than 29,000 people die[1] and 256,000 are seriously hurt in aggravated assaults/ADWs (assaults with a deadly weapon), and who knows how many are raped because of this stupid process. Want to take a guess what it is worldwide? I don't.

Look at "having to win" as a temporary (or sometimes, as in the case of stalkers, permanent) form of insanity. The person becomes so locked in on something he can't see anything else. Normal checks and boundaries just fly out the window. It's the same thinking (or lack thereof) that makes it so that you can't reason with a drunk. The drunk's circuits are temporarily out of commission. The guy is going to keep on pushing it until *he* perceives that he's won. Great; that means you'll be relying on a wacko's perceptions for a braking mechanism. Not in this lifetime, sweetheart.

The answer to "how far can it go" depends on who's involved. If it's only short-term insanity, what he's looking for is a signal that he recognizes as his adversary going belly-up. Hopefully, once he gets that he'll back off. If this is a more permanent form of stupidity, then who knows where it will end. Accept this as gospel here, folks, from someone who's faced these fuckers: *someone who "has to win" will habitually go to extremes that would make all but the most fanatical flinch away, saying, "Whoa! Wait a minute! Too much!"*

In extreme cases, this fixation exists in spite of how much damage the person causes or even what it might cost him to do it! Realize that there are loose cannons out there with the philosophy of "victory at any cost." They go in full bore, and that leaves you facing an overcommitted wacko. What's so scary about dealing with one of these guys is that, while he is not, quote unquote, suicidal, he's only thinking about winning, not necessarily surviving. You need to realize that he is *totally committed*, and all the normal safety checks we rely on other people having are off line.

The ones you're more likely to meet, however, are the people who go retarded temporarily and take on that same attitude long enough to cause some major damage. The guy's got no idea what kind of a can of worms he's opening, yet he's going to come charging on in anyway. The good news is that he's the type who will respond to the gentle forms of persuasion we're going to cover in this book.

Where most of these wankers make a critical mistake (and I'm going to give you a reeeeaaaal big important safety tip here) is *they think that violence is just another stage in the escalation!* WRONG!

Most people look on physical violence as a way to raise the ante in a game of escalato. What they don't realize is that by using physical violence, they've changed the game entirely!

How many fights have you seen where it looked like two people skittering forward, throwing a punch, and then skittering back, hoping that the hurt they inflicted on the other idiot was enough to stop that person from continuing the fight? In many of these situations, the person doing the hurting seemed to be saying to him or herself, "Oooh, I'm scared about being here! I hope this hurts him enough to make him back down," rather than settling down to the job of *really* trying to hurt the other fighter. The thought is to hurt the guy just enough to make him stop so the person can say to himself, "I won!"[2]

This is not how you stop violence. In fact, this sort of shit increases it. You don't stop violence by incrementally increasing the volume!

People who fight like this are often scared and are generally not thinking about what doors they themselves have opened by striking the other person.[3] I got news for you, folks. When the argument becomes physical, you have just crossed a state line, and the laws are different over in these parts.

The reason I say it's a different game is this (and indeed this is one of my infamous "Animal's Laws of Violence"):

ANYTIME YOU STEP INTO THE ARENA OF PHYSICAL VIOLENCE, YOU *HAVE TO ACCEPT* THAT IT MAY NOT END UNTIL EITHER YOU OR YOUR OPPONENT OR MAYBE BOTH ARE DEAD.

I don't care if it's just a warning slap to someone—it can escalate! *Anytime* you are tempted to resort to violence, this is the bottom line: *if you ain't ready to die for it or kill for it, don't do it.*

Gosh, isn't that a warm fuzzy thought?[4] Knowing this fact is also the main difference between what I call amateurs and professionals. An amateur will use violence as another chip in the poker game of escalato; a pro knows and accepts going in that once it becomes physical, you ain't in Kansas no more. Because of that he'll do everything in his power to keep it from crossing that line. But once that line is crossed, he'll try to get the situation back across the line ASAfuckingP! Because he knows he's gambling with his life.

An amateur, however, either hasn't realized this or has ignored it. He's going to strike out at people without any regard to the magnitude of the thunder he could be calling down.

Why? Because:

Escalato and Why You Shouldn't Play

1) He's never really been in a shitstorm and therefore doesn't realize that he can get hurt.
2) He's careful about bullying someone who he thinks won't retaliate.
3) He's so out of touch with everything except his emotions at the moment that he's totally blind to reality (this is usually aided and abetted by drugs, alcohol, and/or neurosis).
4) He's thinking that it will make him "win."

Only a fool uses violence without regard to where it can lead. Because of this lack of awareness, however, most amateurs will see no problem about escalating a situation into violence. It's not that they're competent at violence (far from it); it's just that they're willing to dive in head first which makes them dangerous. Fools rush in where angels say, "Whoooooa . . . hang on here for a minute!"

Next time you get a chance to watch a conflict brewing between others (even a minor one), pull up a chair, crack a beer, and just sit there and watch. Unless one of the participants is extremely adept at conflict (read: knows how to end it), what you're going to see is a rising spiral of escalation where both people are doing things to hurt the other, hoping that it will bring victory.

I swear it will look like one of those betting sessions I described, with each person throwing something in that is designed to convince the other person that the stakes are too high and that he or she should fold because the first person is willing to go "this far." Naturally, the other person responds with the equally intelligent, "Oh yeah? Well I'm willing to go *this* far!"

It will get louder and nastier and meaner and may eventually evolve all the way to violence, with you sitting there drinking beer and cheering. The combatants lose all perspective on the matter and go at each other at an incredibly accelerated rate over something that is usually really stupid and small. Normally, the person who is willing to raise the stakes to the highest level ends up winning, not because he had the best hand, but because he was willing to go *too* far the fastest.

In extreme situations, whatever little thing it started over gets lost in the insanity of winning until it becomes a matter of life and death. I'm talking weapons here. Either in the middle of the fight someone pulls one or one bozo goes out to his car and comes back with a gun and shoots the other dude. Domestic situations are charm stories all their own. The graveyards are filled with people who didn't think that this could happen when they started arguing.

Oftentimes the weapon is pulled as just another level of escalation. ("Oh yeah! Well look how far *I'm* willing to go!") If a sudden bout of common sense doesn't show up in the other dude's yard, prompting him to run like hell, you've got serious injury looming on the horizon.

It is incredible the number of people who will stand there and keep on going with the fight even when the other dude is flashing a weapon. I've heard drunk morons proclaim, "I don't care if he's got a knife!" No lie! The one I couldn't believe was when I heard a real genius proclaim, "You ain't got the balls" to someone wagging a gun around. Guess what? He had the balls.

Now as stupid as the soon-to-be-a-corpse may sound under these conditions, the clown with the weapon is being just as retarded. You'd be shocked at the number of people who get this dumb look on their face when they realize, "Oh my God! I really did hurt him."

Duuuuhhh! If that ain't what you were trying to do, why'd you pull the weapon out? And why are you surprised now that you've succeeded? Hopefully, if a weapon is produced, one person or the other will decide that the stakes have suddenly gotten too high and pull out, or there are other people around who will intercede before the stakes really do get too high. However the yearly body count shows that there's a whole lot of people who don't suffer sudden attacks of common sense. (The German proverb of "when two argue, both are at fault" makes a whole lot more sense in this light, doesn't it?)

Let me state here and now that professionals don't play escalato! Why? Because they know what could be waiting for them across that line in the arena of violence. And they don't want to cross it for no other reason than they've had a bad hair day. Honestly, is that worth dying for? Pros know it could happen.

In my first book I quoted an old-timer as saying, "Violence is the first option and the last choice of the competent." Think about that for a second. It's seriously deep, and it defines the difference between pros and amateurs.

It means pros will not use what they are best at until all the other tools have been exhausted. However, once the decision is reached to employ violence, the amount of destructive energy professionals can and will unleash is awesome to behold.

Why? Because they are not fighting to "win," *they are fighting to end it!*

At first glance that may look to be one in the same thing, but let me tell you they are worlds apart.

Escalato is an ego game. The person who "won" can wander off humming to himself how right he was, etc., etc. Someone who is fighting to end it isn't fighting for warm fuzzies for his ego. He is fighting to get it out of the realm of the physical ASAP because he knows what can and will happen if it goes on too long.

Often, by being a superior force with physical violence, the conflict can and does end quickly. However there is always the possibility that it may not, especially if you're going for victory rather than a quick ending! I've seen and experienced many a supposedly easy victory turn into a serious fur ball of claw and fang because the party went into it with the wrong goal.

That is why it is so important to make one of your primary goals to neutralize the threat! When you do that, you end it. If I drop someone in three moves, it isn't to punish him; it's to keep him from being able to take it into the physical arena again anytime soon. Once I have him back over the line, he's going to know that path is closed to him. When he's lying there hurting from hitting the ground and in a wrist lock, he's going to know that it was a mistake to try to escalate it into violence.

There are other types of escalation than the "I gotta win" type, but this book would turn into an encyclopedia if I tried to explain them all. What's important is to recognize the basic pattern. I've said it before: you don't need to know the type of shark to recognize a shark attack.[5] Go out and watch for these patterns. You'd be amazed at how widespread this behavior is.

ENDNOTES

1. *1993 Uniform Crime Report* (numbers rounded off)

2. When I watch normal people fight, I'm often reminded of what rabbits and kangaroos look like when they box—lots of fists flailing in the middle while both heads are leaning back trying to avoid getting punched in the face.

3. Incidentally, this also applies to rape. You'd be amazed at how many women initiate the actual physical violence. They strike the guy, who was, until then, only a potential assailant. Bam! Escalato! The woman is the one who took it to the physical level. This isn't PC, but unfortunately it's true. *Never* strike someone unless you're willing to take it all the way.

4. Its corollary is, "Don't make it easier to kill you than to leave you alive. You won't like the answer." Another barrel of laughs, eh?

5. In the same vein as you don't need a Ph.D. in ichthyology to recognize a shark attack, you don't need a Ph.D. in psychology to be able to recognize these sorts of patterns.

Gettin' a Move On

CHAPTER 2

Professional Standards

#13 The important things are always simple.
#14 The simplest things are always hard.
#15 The easy way is always mined.
                    —Murphy's Laws of Combat

Now I want to turn your attention from what *not* to do regarding violence to what it takes to become a heavy-level player. The object of the exercise is to not get hurt, not be some sort of kung fu killer superhero. The problem with being a kung fu commando is that you're wired so tight that you become an outcast of society. You're just as likely to go off on a loved one as you are someone who deserves it.

Inherent in the professional level of competence are two factors. One is "awareness"[1] and the other is "the trigger." I want to touch upon the first one briefly and the second one a little more in depth.

As readers of my other books may have noticed, I'm a big fan of awareness. For those of you who've never had to slough through any of my other books, simply stated, awareness is a blend of two things. One is being in touch with your external and internal environment; the second is knowing what things mean in that particular place (sometimes referred to as "knowing how things work 'round here").

The first concept is pretty easy to understand. Don't get so caught up with what's going on inside your head that you fail to see the buffalo stampede coming down on you. If you don't see it coming at all, then there ain't much you can do to prevent it, much less keep your tail from being flattened. If you see it coming, however, you can do something about it or at least get out of the way. In short, pay attention to what's going on around you.

The second part of the first part (is it me or did I just sound like a lawyer?) is, "know thyself." What are your strengths? Your limits? What will you tolerate? What won't you tolerate? What are you like under different conditions? You wouldn't think about flying a plane without knowing the aircraft's limitations and specifications, would you? Then why try to live your life without knowing the same about yourself?

When are you most likely to rip someone's head off for looking at you cross-eyed, and when will you let bloody murder slide? Know where you are and what you're like there. For example, while many people are amazed at how mellow I am when they meet me, there is a reason I'm called Animal. I have a state which I call "FIDO" (Fuck It Drive On) in which I will maul anybody or anything that gets in my way and not even slow down.

I know this about myself, and when I'm heading toward a FIDO mood I clear my table of anything I don't want broken, including people. That way I end up doing a whole lot less apologizing. There has been many a time when I've simply turned and walked away from a situation because I felt Animal rear up inside of me. I do this so I don't lose my cool and let Animal break people, which I will do in that mind-set. Know yourself well enough to recognize when you're heading down a certain path before it's too late to turn aside.

In a related venue, what chemically altered states are you prone to become violent under (and hence should avoid)? I can tell you when my blood sugar drops because I become a wolverine with a toothache. Furthermore, me and Tennessee whiskey don't mix. I avoid putting myself into those states these days.

By knowing these things, I can plan accordingly and give people more slack when my internal thermometer is up. If nothing else, I can warn them and if they persist, then it's on them for not listening. Knowing this about yourself can do wonders for avoiding trouble and keeping you from abusing the information in this book.

The second part of awareness is knowing how things work, both in general and in a particular area. As near as I can tell, what common sense really is is knowing how things work. That means knowing in real life, if you do this, that happens. It's not hypothetical or rhetorical knowledge; it's knowing what my engineer friend meant when he said, "There are certain undeniable basics. We know if we don't do this, the wings will fall off the airplane."

That kind of wisdom comes from having "been there, done that" rather than mental academic gymnastics.[2] Common sense is blending several different things to get an accurate overall picture. For example, when it comes to fighting, it's a blend of physics, psychology, anthropology, physiology, sociology, immediate interpretive awareness, and experience that makes a good fighter, not just training. Pros subconsciously mix these things together to get the kind of awareness I'm talking about.

With this knowledge of how things work comes the dual awareness of, "*This is what I want to do and this is what I don't want to do.*" The latter is not a well-known concept in this culture, as it is from a form of thinking based on negative space,[3] but if your dick is on the line, you'd better pay attention to it.

An example of what you don't want to do is go to Biker

Corner on Hollywood Boulevard in Los Angeles, walk up to a line of motorcycles, and begin to play with one's kickstand to see how it works. That is most definitely a not do!

As obvious as that may sound, you'd be amazed. The guy who actually did that was a Ph.D. and, while he could tell you all about neurological pathways in the brain, he had no clue as to how "things worked" on a social level. He was just interested in the physical design of a kickstand, and scientific interest overruled everything else, including what would be the ramifications of his actions. Once he clicked into this mind state, he just edited out everything else, including the five bikers standing there drinking beer. He got upset when my friend pulled him back from the brink of disaster. This is a perfect example of both types of awareness, or lack thereof. Much trouble can be avoided by knowing how to read the signs of etiquette for where you are.[4]

The other part of this awareness is recognizing where a particular road is heading. When you see the guy start floating toward the realm of violent behavior, he hasn't gotten froggish yet so you can still stop him before he can jump to that lily pad. Once he gets to that stage where he starts thinking about it though, it's your last chance to stop him without violence. There is all sorts of body language you need to learn to recognize the guy getting there if you want to live long enough to finish getting all your gray hairs.[5]

Once you have established a pretty good set of awareness standards, you begin to move over the next phase of this process: the trigger.

Now I thought very carefully about the choice of the word here. (Amazing how sitting back and peeling an orange can be made to sound like profound thinking, eh?)

Remember in Chapter 1 when I discussed how escalato is like a poker game? Well having a trigger is the best way to prevent becoming involved in a game of physical escalato. It's having four aces ready and waiting and then "calling" the second someone tries to raise the stakes to a physical level. There ain't no more escalato—it ends right now.

Basically, a trigger is an automatic reaction to a well-defined set of standards that you have for other people's behavior. To put it another way, it's a conditioned response to known danger signals.

Ready for another one of Animal's important safety tips? One of those things that differentiates the amateurs from the pros? A point so basic that most martial artists forget it the more trained they get? Why the more real-time experienced someone gets, the more they focus on it?

Here it is—before a person physically attacks, two things *have* to happen: he has to make a mental decision to attack, and the command has to be sent to his body.

That's probably one of the biggest "Animal, tell me something new" statements I've ever made. But before you start filing me with the Bruce Tegner books, let me point out that focusing on this process instead of worrying about the guy's actual attack has reduced the the number of times that I've been hit by over 95 percent and has kept nasty sharp things from doing exploratory surgery on me!

If you've ever seen a hard-core old-timer, a vet, or a pro in action, it seems almost psychic the way he knew it was about to go down. At a glance, he knew to clear for action before the guy even got close to him. When it does happen, he's standing there facing the dude one second and the next, WHAM! Game over. Usually it happens so fast that most people have no idea what started it!

(By the way, for the lack of a better word for this kind of fighting, I'm going to call it "quicktime" rather than the other terms I've heard like blitzkrieg fighting, kamikaze fighting, etc. While those may sound more exciting, I fear they miss the point. Realistically, with this kind of violence, you know it's "quicktime" because it's over so fast.)

Wanna know what the pro was doing? He was watching the other guy for the physiological signs that follow the decision to become violent. In other words, he's watching not for the guy's first move but his decision to make a move! If you know what to look for, you can read an antag-

Professional Standards

onist like a book. While the guy's body is busy preparing for violence, the pro just ups and aborts the process for him.

Picture this. You're in an emotional situation. Things aren't going well. Finally you decide, "That's it! This is too much!" With this decision comes the idea that the best and fastest way to solve everything is to just punch the asshole who's giving you trouble. First your mind has to shift gears into a primal mode. Now your body has to prepare for the forthcoming exertion of energy.

All sorts of commands for reshuffling your body go out. Adrenaline has to be dumped into your system. Blood has shunted away from the skin to supply the muscles. Your breathing increases to compensate for the greater demand you're going to be facing. Then, of course, you have to decide what exactly it is you're going to do. Is it an attack right off the bat, or should you do something else first (like get the guy's hand off you)? Once you decide on this, then a message has to be sent to those particular sets of muscles that will carry out your decision. With all of this going on, is it any wonder a pro can see it coming?

No matter who you are or who you're facing or what culture the guy is from, this process remains the same. It's built into us biologically. If a person doesn't have these reactions, he's got a little antenna, green skin, and pointy ears. But if you're facing a human, you can rely on this process happening. All you need to do is get the basics and brush up on the local versions of the signals.

A major difference between a pro and an amateur is what the pro has cued up and waiting on the other side of the decision to become violent. Most people basically have a limp dick waiting, but they're making it up as they go along. Since most violence is sort of whim du jour, they're not likely to be prepared to really rock and roll effectively from the start. Often their first attack is spastic because they didn't have their ducks in line or because they're not sure if they want it to really become violent.

But, given some room to pick up speed, they can and

will run out and get enough bricks to build an effective attack. A pro, on the other hand, already has a ton of bricks waiting to drop on the guy's head the second that line is crossed, and he's already figured out the best place to drop them. Now who do you think is going to win this hand?

Incidentally, for any youngun's out there, here's a free tip. Tune your sensors into exactly how much "weight" there is on the other side of that line. A person with a ton of bricks "feels" different than a dude with an attitude, no matter how pissed he is. It also feels different than someone who is just flat-out crazy enough to shoot you for looking at him. There's a feeling about "heavies" that not only would they be willing to shoot you but they're calm enough about it that they won't miss.

Another thing that makes the pro such a mother to deal with can be found in the statement, "An amateur will look at you and decide *if* he can take you. A pro will look at you and decide *how* to take you."

By that I don't mean he says to himself, "I'm going to use the famous technique of Ichee Ommeee Kazwow (Swooping monkey doing a Tarzan yell by candlelight, a very famous move)". Face it—you can't predict how the other guy is going to move. I know way too many "techniques" that rely on too many specific conditions for them ever to be practical.

What you can do is assess what it is the guy isn't paying attention to. These "holes" in his awareness will indicate what sort of general technique will work best against him. For example, most people do not pay attention to their feet or legs during a fight. This makes them real susceptible to the second basic method to get someone onto the ground: take his support away. Whether it's a heel hook, sweep, trip, check, knee drop, or just busting the dude's knee, that will be decided later depending on how the guy makes his move. All you're doing at this moment is deciding what windows he has left open, hence what you have to do to take him out.

Professional Standards

Most people make the mistake of trying to apply either a specific technique or an overly focused approach to a person's strongest part. That's a waste of time. If the guy's hands are moving too fast and wild, you're not going to be able to get a jujutsu lock on him to take him down, so check out if he's left his support exposed. If so, go after his feet instead. It's quicker and easier, and you're less likely to get hurt than if you tried to force a technique onto a situation.

This is what I mean when I say a pro will know how to take you. He instinctively uses negative-space thinking to decide how to come in on you. He's not coming in where you are, he's coming in where you *aren't*. When he decides to trigger, he already has his target in mind. (See Appendix E.)

By the way, want to know one of the most consistent physiological signs of the decision to become violent? It's an unconscious twitch the entire body undergoes. It looks like a shudder that a person does when he's cold, but just one. His entire body jerks slightly. That twitch means that adrenaline is being dumped into his body preparing for fight or flight. It is accompanied by the guy's skin color changing. The message has been sent, and he's going to move. Once you see this happen, you only have a second to react before he launches his attack, which is why you need to be specifically watching and waiting for that twitch.

In real situations, this jerk can often be covered up by a larger gesture. Watch for that nasty little jerk when someone is yelling, screaming, and waving his arms around. It's subtle, but it'll be there.

A more obvious sign is when it looks like he's taking in a deep breath and suddenly expanding right before he attacks. It ain't no calming breath neither—the guy's anger is swelling up like a balloon about to burst. Still, that twitch and skin color change will be there, often as part of the inhale and puff.

The ones I hate, however, are when the guy suddenly seems to be pulling in, not in submission but like a spring tightening down before it explodes. These guys are like badgers with attitudes, and you shouldn't mess around with them. Those who contract rather than expand are often more experienced and dangerous fighters than puffers. Unlike puffers, who are like bombs going off and affecting anyone nearby, these guys are like howitzers. They're aiming a shell at a specific target. By pulling in, they're toughing up like a hazelnut on steroids, and you just know they're going to be a bear to crack.

There's another type of person you should know about, and he is as bad, if not worse, than the badger. Like the badger, you can recognize him from his reaction to impending violence. When you see this reaction, I don't care who you are—if it goes sideways from that point, you're going to get hurt.

It's when the guy's face goes blank. It is usually accompanied by his eyes going "flat" and his body apparently relaxing. I can't describe it any better than this, but when someone's face goes neutral on you, it means he's just dumped adrenaline into his system but he has enough control to still talk and think. You are now dealing with a combat-ready wolverine that can and will explode on you.

The adrenaline dump is what makes the person go cold. His skin color changes and for the same reasons as other people. If he is standing, his shoulders could drop only a fraction of an inch and his hands will drop to the side. He'll often shift to target you. If he's sitting, he may reposition his body, and that hand that's now on the table or chair arm is going to help him launch at you. Aggressors seriously fuck up when they mistake this neutral ready pose for submissive body language. Nothing could be further from the truth. I've seen serious blood fly over this mistake, and it almost always belonged to the guy who misread the danger signs.

Under these conditions, your best weapon is to *start talking!* Negotiate. Compromise. Apologize. Do whatever it takes, but *stop pushing*. You can still hold the boundries and come to a compromise, but back off on pushing him.

I'm dead serious about how dangerous these guys are. The good news is that they have enough self-control not to just go off on you. The bad news is they have enough self-control to go straight for your throat when they release the dogs of war.

For those of you with a more esoteric bent, I agree that, yes, you can see the dude cross the line in his eyes, even a second or so before the adrenaline dump, but try and explain exactly what it looks like. Pupil contraction? Eye color change? "Hardening" of the eyes? Yeah, but which one signals that the dude just crossed the line? It's there, but unfortunately it's too subtle to explain in a book. But oooh man, you know what it means when you've seen it firsthand.

Incidentally, you won't see these prefight reactions in movies or in sport fights. With the first it's because they're fantasy. (Besides, it takes all day to film a three-minute fight scene. I know; I've worked on martial arts movies.) With the second, the guy is already psyched up to fight, although I've noticed that they sometimes do it when the bell rings for the first round and they come out of their corners.

Now an interesting point should be made here, one that truly differentiates the pros from the tough guys[6] and psychos. *Someone can have lots of experience with violence—in fact, he might even be able to go full bore once he crosses that line—yet still not be a good fighter!*

The reason is, this sort of person is relying not on his skill so much as the effect his attitude is going to have on his victim. In fact, most so-called tough guys rely simply on being more willing to become violent than the person they attack. That, more than anything, carries the day for them.

Why? Because he's still playing escalato! He's learned that by attacking first he can get the upper hand and "win" in most cases. What he's really relying on is not so much his fighting skills as his blitzkrieg to freak out his victim.

Want to know something funny? Most of these guys don't have the vaguest idea what to do if their blitzkrieg attack doesn't work! They rely so much on the attack working that when it doesn't, they're stumped. I've seen guys literally freeze when their attack failed while they decided what to do next. By relying too much on attacking first and overwhelming their victims, these clowns never learned how to fight. They may excel when it comes to beating people up, but that isn't fighting.

If you not only survive their blitz but bring one right back at them, they're in some deep kimchee![7] Blowing up fast and winning fast, as these guys do, is neither fighting nor being tough. It's being an aggressor. If this sounds like an extreme case of bullying, that's because it is! What he's doing is an assault, not a fight. It's when they mess up and tree themselves a bad one that they discover just exactly how unskilled at war they are.

The same thing often happens with drunks and those who have little experience in fighting. I cannot begin to tell you the number of dumb looks I've seen by simply leaning back and letting a guy's fist fly past my face. Of all the reactions the dude was expecting, me getting out of the way wasn't one of them. It doesn't mean that once he gets it together he's not going to attack again, but that split second of "DUH" is a moment you can exploit to your advantage.

A trigger is knowing what the build-up to violence looks like and having your bricks, blueprints, and construction crew waiting just the other side of the line if he decides to get froggish. In other words, anytime someone tries to take it to a physical level, you *immediately* do whatever you physically have to do to end it before he can pick up any more steam.

Do you know why you have to do this? Because the farther out past the line of violence he goes, the harder it's going to be for you to stop the violence! And if you don't stop it immediately, he's going to pick up more speed. The faster he's going and the farther out he gets, the more dangerous he is.

So how do you stop a physical attack? By being better at physical violence than the other guy! There is no other way to derail the process once it has started. You are going to have to hurt him sufficiently to snap him out of both the violence itself and the mental state that created it. Now, until he actually attacks you can try to use other tools (and maybe they'll work), but once he crosses that line and commits to an attack, end it!

You have to become physical in order not to get hurt. You have to do it immediately. And you have to land on him hard enough to convince him to stop. The farther gone he is, the harder you're going to have to land on him. He needs to know that crossing that line with you was a serious mistake. If he doesn't learn this immediately, he's going to keep on trying!

By laying down a serious wad all at once, you avoid the nickel-dime game of escalato most people play. This is something that those yo-yo social reformers and the American Civil Liberty Naz . . . uh . . . Union are missing. Trying to "contain" someone in a violent state will only escalate it! If you try to contain someone without hurting him, he is going to react to it as another chip in the escalato process. There are physiological reasons for this, which I will explain in the next chapter.

Again, your "trigger" means anytime someone tries to offer you physical violence, you immediately land on him with whatever level of violence is appropriate to end it. Once physical violence is introduced, this program kicks in automatically. It's like a real trigger—once it is pulled, it sets off an automatic response and something nasty is going to follow less than a second later. No "homina homina homina, oh me, is this real violence? What should I do about it?" etc., ad nauseam.

Change your thinking about this. You're not there to win a fight or even to get the guy to back down. Your only goal is to END VIOLENCE IMMEDIATELY! This more than anything else will start you along the path to developing your trigger. The other part is chaining your awareness to your reactions and vice versa. To know is to act. (This also helps prevent accidental discharge, which is a book unto itself.) Then it's just a matter of practice.

It sounds paradoxical, but once you enter this level of thinking, 90 percent of all the trouble that was out there

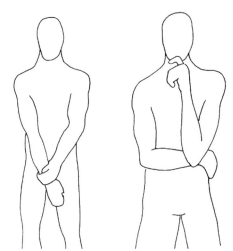

Figure 1. Note that these two ready stances are not normal fighting stances. However from each of these positions you can flow immediately into either attack or defense. Also, both of them are designed to protect important things you may have grown attached to.

before will choose to pass you by. Without sounding too woo-woo about it, there is just something about people who have triggers that makes the average trouble hunter instinctively look elsewhere for their fun and games. Knowing how to spot this is a matter of life and death to them, and all but the youngest, dumbest, and most psychotic realize it.

That, by the way, is half of the battle on your part. The simple willingness to commit violence is not the same thing as being calmly ready to commit violence. One is a whole lot scarier. Lots of people are willing, but few people show up for class prepared. If you're calmly sitting there with your lesson plan ready, that's going to have a major effect on the outcome of the situation . . . most especially if it will turn violent at all!

What I'm saying is, your preparedness will be sensed by the other players. It shows them that you're there and waiting for them to get froggish. None but the most dumb/drunk/young think they can outdraw and outshoot someone who's got the drop on them. They're thinking about getting stupid, but you're prepared to handle it if they do. I think the word "deterrent" comes to mind here.

Now I must tell you that the trigger is not a toy. With it comes a great responsibility—not misusing it. That means no matter how tired, cranky, stoned, drunk, or just pissed off you may be, you're going to have to develop some serious morals about how and when you use violence. I'd highly recommend that, almost the very second you manage to access your trigger, you spend serious time working with anger management programs. It will save you a shit load of grief in your life if you do.

ENDNOTES

1. For my old readers: Thought I wouldn't manage to slip that one in this book, didn't you? Ha!

2. I recently reread Louie L'Amour's *Education of a Wandering Man*. I highly recommend you spend a few days reading it.

3. What's not there is just as important as what is there. For example, when someone tells you something, ask yourself two questions: "What isn't this person telling me about this situation," and "What's he getting out of telling me this?" Looking for what isn't there (or being mentioned) in a situation can go so far as to save your life.

4. Of course if you want to contribute to my retirement fund, there is always my book *Violence, Blunders, and Fractured Jaws*, which covers in depth how to read your local environment.

5. Not only do I recommend my video *Safe in the Street*, but I highly recommend the book *Manwatching* by Desmond Morris, or spend a few weekends watching Morris' "The Human Animal" series on The Learning Channel (TLC).

6. Wannabe tough guys, that is. After all, these "tough guys" aren't that tough!

7. You'd be amazed at how many of today's gangbangers can't fight their way out of paper bag. They can and will shoot you in a second, but if you catch them without a weapon or move on them before they can get it out, it's amazing how fast they go down.

CHAPTER 3

Physiology, Psychology, and Other Mumbo Jumbo

---

1) Never make a plan without knowing as much as you can about your enemy.
2) Never be afraid to change your plans when you receive new information.
3) Never believe you know everything.
4) Never wait to know everything.

—Robert Jordan
Lord of Chaos

T up and I were only about a hundred yards away when McQueen's voice crackled over the radio: "KNIFE!" The radio became ominously silent after that one word. We'd been moving toward the trouble to assist, but after hearing this we broke into a dead run.

As we ran, I handed off my radio to Tup. He was the reasonable end of the two of us; this was my department. Since we had been closest we were the first to arrive on the scene.

We stopped running and looked down at McQueen and his attacker. The knife-wielding assailant was sitting on the ground with his legs out in front of him, obviously having been knocked over onto his butt. McQueen was kneeling in front of him, right arm around the dude's neck in a chokehold kinda thing. The guy's head was tucked against his chest. With his left hand, McQueen was easily fending off the dude's feeble attempts to hit him. Laughing boy was curled up, locked up, and not going nowhere.

"Got him?" I asked tensely, ready to jump into it.[1]

"Yeah," he grunted back as the rest of the troops arrived.

With that I relaxed and began to look carefully at what exactly was going on.

Now it didn't take a rocket scientist to figure out who had gotten the best of this situation. However, we weren't dealing with a rocket scientist.

"Let me up motherfucker! I'll kick your ass!"

All evidence to the contrary. Never mind the lack of logic on this assertion. But then again, Mr. IQ wasn't real logical at the moment. He was sitting there threatening someone who had not only just disarmed him but dropped him onto the ground and then locked him up. But did that matter? Noooo! When he got free he was gonna kick some ass.

A few goons arrived and stepped up to help. Imagine the offensive line of the San Francisco 49ers on a bad hair day. Them kind of guys made up the goons. While I'm an old kneecap buster from way back, I would've had to climb a stepladder to reach some of these guys' knees. When they went to town, I made it a habit to get out of their way so I wouldn't get stepped on accidentally.[2] With the cavalry there, Tup and I started looking around for the knife, which had been smacked off somewhere into the bushes. (Never did find the friggin' thing.)

I heard McQueen tell the guy that he was going to let him go and that he was to lie back down on the grass. I thought to myself, "Mistake. He ain't ready."

Sure enough, when released from the headlock, Chuckles tried to go ballistic again. Fortunately there were about three goons waiting for him. The guy lay down—not quietly, and not without help—but lay down he did. Ten minutes or so later, they took him away. He was still mouthing off, but he had cooled off enough to realize that he was seriously outgunned.

All in all, that whole situation was dealt with in about 20 minutes and took about 10 guys total. At no time did anyone use excessive force and, while it wasn't exactly a proscribed takedown, it got him down and controlled without damaging him. It was a good, clean, by-the-book process. In other words, "no blood, no foul" and, best of all, no lawyers.

Which is great, if you got them kind of resources available. However, unless you're a member of the local police department or security team complete with radio backup, the odds are you aren't going to have that sort of help when it all goes south. And, even if you are a member of the aforementioned, the odds are that when it comes at you in the dark, you're going to have to handle it alone until backup can arrive. Tup and I got there in less than a minute from the call, but a guy with a knife can do a lot of damage in less than a minute.

The reason I knew that guy wasn't ready to be let go was because *he still had an attitude!* And it was the wrong one! Once the constraints were removed, what did he try to do? Continue fighting! Sorry, chump; wrong answer. Since he still had an attitude, they were obliged to fight him back down into a different form of restraint.

That is why I would like to take this opportunity to introduce a concept that I call "Attitude Interrupter." It's a useful little tool that I'm sure you'll find many swell uses for. In fact, most experienced fighters already have one or two, but this tool is sooooo useful you'll probably want dozens of them for various occasions.

An Attitude Interrupter, or AI, is something that makes the guy quit thinking about what he's going on about and

Physiology, Psychology, and Other Mumbo Jumbo

start thinking about a more pressing issue—namely, the pain that your popping him one has caused him. And this new issue ain't no gentle raptaptapping on the window of his conscious. No, the Raven's message is, *I'm in serious pain!* Not the kind of pain that gets people mad, but the kind of pain where you just want to curl up and whimper. This sort of "interrupts" his train of thought. In fact, when the AI is done right, 99 times out of 100 the aggressor suddenly loses any and all interest in fighting. And the good news is it is possible to inflict this kind of pain without permanent damage.

My psychiatrist friends call this sort of behavior "pattern interruption." It's where you take a person's mental program and derail it. What AIs do is give someone stimuli that is so off the track from the one that the guy is running along that the dude goes "huh?" and basically trips himself mentally.[3] Then, with the "therapist's" help, he begins to analyze his actions and emotions from a rational, more functional viewpoint.

From here the person can now understand that, while his emotional reaction may have been very real, it was not actually in accord with reality around him. This brings him back from listing so far to starboard to a more even keel, commonly called "normal" by those of us not in the psychiatric world.

Incidentally, I highly recommend you look into the concept of pattern interruption (try the book *Emotional Intelligence* by Daniel Goleman), as it is a fantastic way to stop escalating problems in their tracks without the use of violence. I know of one incident where a drug freak with a knife who'd been holding off 10 people was disarmed by a naked woman who just walked up to the guy. He spun around and threatened her with it, screaming, "Do you want this," and she held out her hand and calmly said, "Yes." Her response and state of undress caught the dude so off guard he just handed her the knife. Free sneaky trick there for those of you who want to use it. (I'm talking about pattern interruptions, not trying to disarm people when you're naked . . . although come to think of it, I've done that too.)

While pattern interruption may make the guy trip himself mentally, AIs are for when you want to derail the train for him! While he's trying to figure out what's going on, you use that period of time to your advantage. In other words, while he's going "huh?" you land on him and make sure he ain't getting up anytime soon.

Look at it this way. Most people in the middle of a freak-out, argument, or drunk are more wrapped up with what is going on inside their own head than what's going on around them. What they don't see is the damage they're causing or the stupidity of their actions. See, their emotional state is what is running their actions, and until you get them out of that territory, they're going to continue to flip out on you. Generally, it's going to get worse before it gets better.

As long as that internal message is louder than anything else, that's what he's going to be hearing. This is why when it's still nonviolent, normal pattern interruption is such a useful tool. It double clutches the guy's spinout, and while he's considering what to do next he's fundamentally shut down for a time. While the person is frozen and going "homina homina homina," the psychiatrist makes his move.

When it becomes physical, then you use an Attitude Interrupter for the same purpose. You send in a different message than what he expected, and while he's chewing it over, you make your move. By using an AI you open the door again for the sweet song of reason. Of course the kind of reason we're talking about is, "You fucked up asshole. Now shut up, sit down, and do what I tell you or I'll mop the floor with your face!" (But that's reasonable, isn't it?)

So an Attitude Interrupter is a deliberate, painful, and nasty move that is several things at once.

One, it's an interruption of the mental process that is causing the person to misbehave.

Physiology, Psychology, and Other Mumbo Jumbo

Two, it causes a moment of hesitation, which is your window of opportunity to put him into one of those nice, neat takedown/holds that people who've never actually dealt with violence love to tell you is how you should do your job.

Three, it's an immediate punishment for him escalating the situation to a physical level. He took it over the line, and this is what it costs for doing that. It don't matter how he acts around others, he doesn't pull that shit with you. By being immediate, it lets him know where he stands with you. That kind of dog pack mentality is generally understood by people who use physical violence.[4]

Four, it's a warning to him that he'd better cool it now, because you can, and will, do a whole lot worse if he keeps it up. Granted the dude may start mouthing, but the odds are he's not going to try and take it physical again.

Five, it's knowing how to inflict painful, but not necessarily damaging, actions. A well-placed uppercut to the diaphragm can be more effective at stopping someone than a five-cell flashlight across the head. Best of all, it's harder to get called onto the mat (or get sued) for the former.

Now let me tell you what happens if you don't use Attitude Interrupters and just try to control the guy physically. The message that he chose to mess with the wrong dude *does not get delivered*. Even if you take him down to the ground in some fancy dan jujutsu move, the idiot will still want to fight you! Remember that stupid game of escalato? He's going to be trying to raise the stakes until you wake him up to the following points: A) this is not a game, B) he better start paying attention to what's actually going on around him, and C) it's him that's going to come out on the short end.

I have seen guys pick themselves up from judo throws and think they fell down! They didn't realize that what had just happened wasn't an accident and that they were up against a skilled fighter. In the same vein, look at the guy at the beginning of this chapter. His knife taken away, him knocked down and locked up, surrounded by 10 guys, and he still thought he had a chance of winning. Remember, the guy is in a state of stupid to begin with, so his making more stupid decisions shouldn't surprise you.

What's worse, without an AI, the sucker is going to come up from the ground even madder than before! The minor amount of pain he received from just being taken down has only served to infuriate him and spur him on, not overwhelm his internal responses.

I cannot begin to tell you how true this is. I've not only faced it many times, but I've seen it countless times more. Anyone who's ever had to do a proscribed takedown[5] on someone can tell you that they often do not put an end to the situation. If you don't interrupt his attitude, the guy goes more ballistic over being restrained until he either exhausts himself or escalates it to the point where you do have to hurt him. Generally in these situations, you end up hurting the guy much worse while trying to restrain him than if you had just slammed him with an AI up front.

There is one very important point about using AIs. ONCE YOU'VE LAID ONE OR TWO INTO THE DUDE AND YOU'VE GOTTEN HIM DOWN, DON'T DO ANOTHER ONE. You can really step on your dick with one if you're not careful. As extreme as the situation is, there still is a fine balance between what you need to do to control him and the use of excessive force.

With physical force, there is a point where, by AIing the guy, then dropping him and controlling him, you've established dominance. He's laying there more concerned about moaning than fighting. On the other side, if you keep on inflicting pain once the guy is down and controlled, he's going to fight you just to protect himself. As far as he's concerned, you're telling him to sit still and you're continuing to hurt him. Under those conditions it's natural for him to try and fight back. This is often real difficult to figure out in the middle of the whole furball, but it's important.

Once you have the guy down on the ground and locked up, your goal is to keep it from going back over the line into violence. You are now the barrier preventing him from going over that line again. From here on, your mouth is your greatest weapon for controlling him, not your grip. Do what you have to do to control the guy, but remember: odds are you're pumped on adrenaline yourself, so you might be adding a little more pressure on the hold than you need to. Remember *awareness of self*. It is important.

There's another point that needs to be considered, especially with street people. Until the Gracie brothers showed the martial arts world that fights often go to the ground (even if they had to take it there themselves to prove their point), most people thought that fights were only fought on one's feet. Once one guy went to the ground and decided to stay there, supposedly the fight was over. Everyone knows who's the top dog. He's down, you stop attacking and go pee on a tree. It has to do with this whole dominance and submission thing (like why kings, priests, and judges are seated higher than anyone else in the room).

You'll notice I say "most people." Here's a problem. Street people know that going to the floor is a death sentence or, at the very least, a trip to the hospital. Anyone on the ground runs the risk of being stomped to death not only by the attacker but by the onlookers. A street person, therefore, is going to do anything and everything in his power to get up until you convince him that you're not playing by the street rules. In other words, contrary to what he thinks, his only chance of *not* getting hurt is to stay down!

Under these circumstances you really have to lay a serious AI on the dude up front, lock him up, and then start talking. His every instinct is going to be bucking against him staying down and still. You gotta show him that only by staying down and still (read: passive) can he hope not to receive any more pain.

Now for those of you who are interested, besides the psychological reason there's a solid physiological reason why you need to use AIs. (For those of you not interested, just skip ahead to the murder and mayhem part of this book, but if you ever think you're going to have to explain in court why you had to hit the guy so hard, you may want to stick around and practice your self-defense plea.) It has to do with how our nervous system works—or, more specifically, doesn't work—under high-stress situations.

The human nervous system can only handle so much information at once. This is a physical limitation having nothing to do with psychology. It has to do with how much juice can pass down a certain gauge wire at any one time. Whatever you want to call it, the baud rate, amplitude, p.s.i. tolerance, whatever, in our physical nervous system is only so much. Once we reach that level, the system shuts off extraneous signals that are not relevant to the main message. Once this happens, the only kind of message that is going to get through is one that is *louder* than all the rest.

The more intense the situation is, the more unrelated stuff gets edited. Stuff like higher brain functions, for example! When those go, the normal checks and balances that allow us to function in society go *pffffft*.

As the guy advances down the path of unreason, more and more stuff has to get edited. His system is running full speed ahead, fixating on whatever has got his panties in a wad. In order to keep this fixation up, he has to drop more and more subroutines and mental functions until eventually the guy is totally focused on being bent out of shape. I probably don't have to mention that by this time, little things like logic, reason, concern that he's being a total asshole, social restriction against using violence, and so forth are all stashed in a dusty, unused corner of the warehouse of his mind.

An AI jolts his nervous system out of freakout mode by injecting a louder set of messages. It's like whacking a TV to bring it back into focus. It causes the circuits to start behaving the way they're supposed to. If it doesn't, then your dealing with something worse than just a loose wire.

All of this can be complicated by several things. The worst is the physical effects of alcohol. Now while I have seen a few fights go down while everyone was sober, I think it would be safe to say that a majority of the violence I have seen involved one, both, or all people under the influence of alcohol and/or drugs. Guess what alcohol does to your central nervous system? That's right! It shuts down the higher brain functions. The neural pathways are physically shut down! You try to dial up common sense and you're going to get, "The number you have reached is temporarily disconnected." This is, by the way, why it's true that "you can't reason with a drunk." His reason is gone. (You can, however, lie to, trick, and con one. Handy thing to know.[6])

For those of you who are interested, I've included an appendix on the stages of intoxication. It's important to know these stages if you want to do the right thing when dealing with drunks. I first learned the need for AIs dealing with drunks. Their thought processes are more impeded than people who're just on an emotional freak, so the message has got to be louder.

Incidentally, here's something that I've noticed. I can't prove it, and there's no scientific explanation for it that I've heard, but I do know that other people have noticed it too. That is, different types of alcohol cause different kinds of "drunks." Not only do different types of booze seem to affect how likely a person is to go off, but they also seem to affect *how* they'll go off.

It seems that any way you cut it, whiskey is a mean drunk. Tequila is mercurial (either happy or mean). Wine is passionate (read: emotional). Beer is a slow burn—they're slow to go off, but when they do it's big. As near as I (or the best brains I can find) can figure, it's the different alkaloids in each type of alcohol that have a secondary effect on the brain. I don't know, it may be a myth, but watch for it.

If I may I'd like to change the subject to something else at this time. Face it guys, we have chosen professions that no sane person would ever dream of doing. As a professional bouncer, security team member, bodyguard, orderly, or anyone who faces violence as a part of the job, every day can put us in severe danger. Did you know that there are people out there with guns and knives who have no hesitation about using them? AND IT'S OUR JOB TO TELL THEM THEY CAN'T! "Excuse me, Mr. Attila, I'm sorry but you can't go looting and pillaging today."

It takes a certain type of person with specialized instincts to survive in such an environment. One of the most important of these instincts is the ability to recognize when you've got a rough one and what you're going to have to do to come out with even a semblance of being intact. In other words, "Bubba, ya gotta know when you done treed yourself a bad one."

As a professional, much of your job is that you have to land on trouble and contain it. Containing someone takes a whole lot more skill than just dropping him. When you're talking about your average obnoxious drunk or street skell, this is pretty easy to do. There are more people out there who are incompetent with violence than competent. So it's not unreasonable to think that this should work under a majority of circumstances.

The real disadvantage is that no matter what circumstances you do this under, the fact that you're dealing with violence perhaps on a daily basis seriously ups your chances of getting hurt. No matter how good you are, even a street skell can still get in a lucky shot. (Remember Murphy and that damned law of his?) And you can't just crush the guy's skull to make sure he doesn't get a piece out of you. This is a serious drawback to your chosen profession.

Now comes the real issue. If the dude is good, I don't care how good you are, you're going to get torn up. If the dude is real good (or seriously flipping out), you're going to have to drop him! There is no safe way to contain someone who is of equal or greater skill than you, especially if his goal is to hurt you. I don't care what any lawyer or martial artist says about this, I'm talking real life here. Even Royce Gracie got mauled in Ultimate #4.[7] He won, but he got torn up so badly that he couldn't continue. That's called a Pyrrhic victory. (Go look

Physiology, Psychology, and Other Mumbo Jumbo

that phrase up; it's an important reality break.) I don't believe in Pyrrhic victories. A head-on with someone who's as dangerous as yourself results in the old Chinese saying, "When two tigers fight, one dies, the other is wounded."

But now our lives are made more difficult by backseat drivers—scum-sucking lawyers, unreasonable employers, sanctimonious members of the press, naive citizens, bleeding-heart liberals, social reformers, and any asshole with a line of rhetoric and an ax to grind. These people—without the benefit of ever having had to wrestle a crackhead down to the ground themselves—tell us that we have to use those same techniques that we use on the minor leaguers *in every situation*. The thinking behind this is, "You're professionals. You should be able to do this easily." Even when we "professionals" realize that somebody is a real bad one and if we just shoot the guy we could save ourselves loads of trouble, policy is more concerned with protecting the company rather than your or my ass.

This brings up a bit of a dilemma. Should I sacrifice myself for the legal protection of the whole, or should I stay alive and make work for lawyers? Well I've always maintained that I like work (I can watch it for hours), so let's make some lawyers sweat for their paychecks.

As a professional you'll need two triggers. The first activates the quicktime program to end violence by controlling the troublemaker. This is not a kill switch! It is quicktime, but when you move you're doing three things:

1) You're preventing him from further violent action.
2) You're containing him in such a way that you don't do permanent damage.
3) You're AIing the SOB to help you achieve the first two.

The second trigger is what most people would think of as a first trigger. This you reserve for when you've looked at the situation and realized there is just no way that the first trigger is going to work. With this trigger you just go into straight-out combat mode. You don't even try to control the dude. When he attacks you, just drop him by any means possible. Reserve this trigger for hard-core attacks, maniacs, and trained/experienced attackers.[8]

There are a couple of reasons why it's important for pros to have these two separate triggers. It establishes reasonable pre-existing standards within yourself with which to gauge any situation you find yourself in. It will also keep you from using excessive force on some obnoxious twerp and getting yourself and the organization you're associated with sued.

Specifically, the first trigger will keep you from going ballistic on some dickweed and possibly killing him. (Maybe not intentionally, but remember Murphy. He's out there waiting.) When you activate this trigger, you know what your goal is going in.

The second trigger will keep you from making a mistake and trying to contain a wolverine on steroids instead of just shooting him, thereby minimizing the amount of blood it's going to cost you for locking horns with Señor Psycho. Mind you, I didn't say it's going to keep you from bleeding. One way or the other, locking up with this kind of fucker is going to cost you.

Like I said, if you're smart you'll keep violence as brief as possible. And for God's sake keep your shit wired tight afterward. This is real life. People who lose fights and are still playing escalato will back up on you, and they often bring weapons!

ENDNOTES

1. Unless it has obviously gone to hell in a handbasket, always check before jumping into a situation like this. If you don't, your interference might just end up being the thing that lets the worm free.

2. The goons were never really sure about me. I was too goofy to be friends with them, but I was also too dangerous for them to object to my goofy behavior. For the most part, we just ended up ignoring each other.

Physiology, Psychology, and Other Mumbo Jumbo

3. If you've ever encountered something so out of the ordinary that you've just stopped and gone "huh?" that's close.

4. I should warn you, however, it is not understood by those who use words as weapons.

5. One of those moves where you're supposed to take the guy down to the ground and restrain him without hurting him so you don't violate his civil rights.

6. Once, out of sheer evil, I conned a drunk who was looking for a fight because we'd cut him off to march down to the state capitol to complain about the liquor laws. I stood at the door of the topless bar smiling and waving as he wobbled off toward downtown.

7. The Ultimate Fighting Championship is the closest thing to real fighting I've seen the martial arts world involve itself in, but until they include guns, knives, and beer bottles and do it on concrete, it's still not there yet.

8. Go watch my video *Winning a Street Knife Fight* to see what constitutes the difference between a correct attack and an incorrect attack. Anyone who attacks you correctly is not someone you can mess around with. They are just too stone-cold dangerous.

Gettin' a Move On

If the enemy is in range, SO ARE YOU!
—Murphy's Law of Combat #20

Before I start this chapter, I want you to do something. Stand up, stay still for a second, and then take a step. Just one step. While you're doing that, I want you to pay attention to what is going on with your body. The reason for this is that what you're going to learn in this chapter is about as difficult as taking a step (in fact, it's sort of the same thing). If you can walk, you can do what I'm going to describe. If you can chew gum at the same time, you can become a grand master.

Well now, boys and girls, I'm about to give you one of those little points that is actually one of the fundamental laws of fighting. It's a little secret that nobody mentions until you've spent about five years in the arts (unless you're reeeeaaaal lucky and have a great teacher or stumbled into a style that teaches it up front). By that time you sort of figure it out by yourself. Oddly enough, this secret is based on something so basic that most people don't even consciously think about it.

So let me ask you a question:

Other than the desire to get laid, what force is pressing on you every moment of your life?

For those of you who said gravity, give yourself a cigar. For those of you who couldn't think of anything other than getting laid, while I understand your response, that is *not* the answer!

Guess what? Gravity is there keeping you from floating out into space every moment of your life. The fact that you are not floating out past Mars proves it (unless of course it was some goooood stuff). Now if that is the case, in which direction does gravity "push" on you? Down. In other words, there is always a downward pressing force on you. Interesting, though not real useful yet, but it will be, especially when you consider the next issue.

Let me ask you another question. Which is faster: muscling something into motion or letting it fall?

For those of you who said letting it fall, that's right! It is faster just to let something head toward the earth than it is to try and shove it along.

Gravity is the fastest and most effective way to get your entire body weight in motion! That's right. You can move faster by intentionally falling down than you can by trying to muscle your weight out of the way. Why? Because gravity is always there pushing down against you! It's not a matter of having to do something, it's a matter of *stopping* doing something. In this case, it's just a matter of you not fighting gravity for a second and nature taking it's course. In other words, you'll start moving.

Where all of this ties in is, all the best fighters utilize their body weight behind their strikes! No weight behind it, wimpy strike. Pretty simple, eh?

Try this. Stand up. Now try throwing yourself to the side. Yeah, just bunny hop to the left or right. Okay, now try lift-

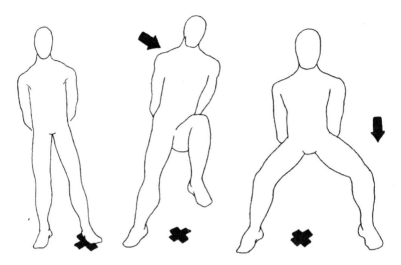

Figure 2. The drop step.

ing just one leg without keeping your balance, like in Figure 2. Whoop! Over you go. Seriously, get up and try this. I'll wait. Besides, I gotta change the CD . . .

Believe it or not, if you did the smart thing and immediately caught yourself before you sucked carpet, you now have discovered the "great secret" of fighting I was just talking about. Yep, y'all is now kung fu grand masters. (Go ahead and start your own style, everyone else does.) The great secret is *letting gravity do your work for you via the controlled fall.* It's called a drop step. Now while this may not sound like much right now, let me tell you that it is the basis of some of the fastest, deadliest, and most devastating fighting techniques that you will ever learn!

Why? First off, it's less work. Generally speaking, that which is less work is faster. Secondly, in less than half a second you managed to get your entire body mass in motion. That means, from a defensive standpoint, you ain't where the fool is attacking anymore. You is gone! Vamoose! Out of the way! Hard to get hurt if you ain't there, now isn't it?

Also consider this. If a guy is throwing a punch at you, which is faster: going "oh no!" and trying to get your arms into defensive position and then throwing yourself to the side, or just falling over and getting your hands up there as backup on your way down? (Yes, it is a trick question.)

From an offensive standpoint, now that your entire body weight is chugging along anyway, why not utilize it to deliver a motherin' powerful blow? You got it! Use it! You can deliver a Nighty Nite Bunny Rabbit in the same time it takes most people to launch and land a setup punch, so why not?[1]

Now remember at the beginning of this chapter when I said that if you can walk you can do this kind of move? Guess what—I wasn't lying. Stand up and walk across the room. Pay attention to exactly what is happening with your body. To walk forward, you shift your balance so you begin to fall, then you push off with your back leg. Then you catch yourself with your other leg. Then you repeat the process. Does this falling, propelling, and catching routine sound vaguely familiar? The reason a drop step is so fast

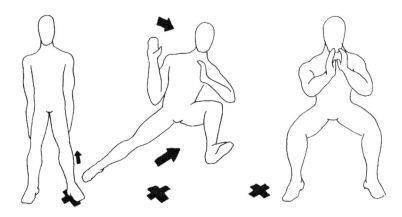

Figure 3. Drop step with spring. Without shifting your weight to regain balance (the natural reaction), just lift your leg and start to fall. Add in the push off from your back leg. Although you'll need less energy because you're already moving, you can move up to three feet this way if pressed. The leg you lifted becomes your landing leg, halting your downward fall.

and effective is because all it is is exaggerated walking! You know how to walk, so you can do this! (And for those of you up to an intellectual challenge, there's a piece of gum taped to the back cover . . .)

Want to make the whole thing faster? Instead of just stepping, throw in the bunny hop you did earlier. That way not only are you falling but you're actively kicking off into the fall by pushing off with your other leg. Look at Figure 3, then give it a shot and see how fast you can go. Just fold one leg up and push into the same direction that you're falling with your other leg. Yeeha!

Here's where it gets real sneaky. Put in the centerline pivot I've described elsewhere[2] and you can go anywhere instantly! Start by folding your leg, then as you're springing, twist in whichever direction you want to go. (Remember to lift your heel so you're springing from the ball of your foot.)

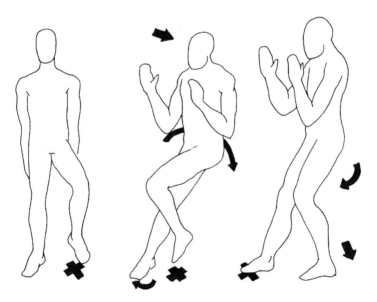

Figure 4. Drop step with pivot. Notice the distance this simple move can cover, and all in under a second. Practice it! Practice it! Practice it! Now the question is, what are you gonna do with such a neat thing? Hang on, we'll go into that in a bit.

Gettin' a Move On

Notice that whatever target on your body someone might have been aiming for is no longer anywhere near its starting point. I would like to point out that it's real hard for most people to change the direction of their attack once it's initiated. (I have a scar on my knuckle from someone who ducked one of my punches in front of a window.) In a nutshell, you've just made his entire attack totally useless! That's safety! It's like Winston Churchill said, "Nothing in life is so exhilarating as to be shot at without result."

After doing that a few times, you'll probably have noticed something. By the time you get your foot back in place to catch you, you've dropped a few inches. (Look at your knees. They're bent now. First hint.) That's just part of the process of doing a controlled fall. Well, what the hell; since it's there anyway, whaddya say we harness it? You can use this lowering process in a few ways.

You can drag your opponent down by attaching your falling body weight to his scrawny ass and watch him go "Aeeeeiii!" as he falls over forward. Or you could slam your weight against his center of gravity/line of stance integrity and watch him go "Aeeeeiii!" as he falls over backward. Or you could put all that juice into an open-handed strike and watch him go "gurgle" and hopefully fall down. Or you could have oodles of fun by combining two of these options and watching all his funny reactions as he realizes something has just gone horribly wrong.

FYI, the combination is the most effective in the long run. The reason is that the combination of a well-placed Nighty Nite Bunny Rabbit and throwing him on his head serves as a great Attitude Interrupter and usually ends the conflict. Think about it. The guy has just had two or more serious AIs laid on his ass (whatever you put on him on the way down plus slamming into the earth). If he's on the floor he's not much of a threat. Not only is he down, but even if he isn't out, if you did it right it's waaaaaay too much work to get back up again and continue hostilities. I've been slammed like this before and let me tell you, I cheerfully volunteered to stay down and inspect the floor when it happened.

Now while options abound as to how to achieve all of these nasty tricks, for the rest of this chapter we're going to focus on striking. Since you're already moving your entire body weight, we might as well use it to ring the guy's chimes.

At this time I seriously want to recommend that you go out and read my book *Fists, Wits, and a Wicked Right* and/or any other book on physiology, fighting targets, pressure points, etc., that you can lay your hands on. The reason is that a well-placed hard blow is ten times more effective than a sloppily placed hard blow. In fact, three well-placed hard blows are more effective than ten equally hard blows scattered wildly around your opponent.[3] The same blow that bounces off a guy's face will break his collarbone. Both will hurt him, but one is more likely to stop him (especially if he has to try to get up off the floor a few seconds later).

I cannot stress enough: *targeting is of utmost importance*. No matter how much oomph you've got, massive firepower not directed correctly is a waste of time. To quote Gordon R. Dickson, "A man with a crossbow in the proper place at the proper time's worth a corps of heavy artillery half an hour late and ten miles down the road from where it should be."[4] While I agree with that, if you use your artillery with the same accuracy that you'd use a crossbow, you're going to be pure hell to tangle with. The kind of blow you're going to be throwing with this move is artillery, but you still have to be accurate to be effective. The same blow that was useless against a guy's chest will blow all the air out of his lungs if delivered eight inches lower and as an uppercut. If he can't breathe he ain't too likely to want to fight, now is he?

I'm going to get Chinese here for a moment. A long time ago in China there was an archery contest. It had been narrowed down to the three greatest archers in the country. The target was fish. (Hey I don't know why, but it was fish, okay?) The archers let fly from a great distance, and all the arrows struck the head near the eye. When the judges asked each of the archers what they were aiming at, the first replied "the fish," the second replied "the head," and the third said "the eye." He won.

In your practice, always "aim for the eye." Don't just try to hit the bag or your opponent; always aim for something specific. On the bag, aim for a stain or spot (even if you have to make one). If you spar, aim for the spots right next to your opponent's tender spots (you don't want to hurt the guy). Under all conditions, don't *ever* just throw a punch, kick, slap, knee, or elbow without a specific target in mind. Even if you miss your exact target, you're going to be a whole lot more focused with your attack. You will discover that one of the key components to quicktime fighting is exactly this kind of control and focus.

In my prime (oh so many beers . . . er . . . years ago), at a dead run I could slam a knife point into an eye-sized target. You could call which eye while I was in flight. Now while that was a while ago, and I'm nowhere near as physically fit as I was back then, that kind of focus left me with an awareness that is a key to quicktime fighting. By aiming at such minute targets in practice, in real fights I increased the number of potential targets on my opponent. The more I focused on precise targeting, the more holes opened in the guy's defenses for me to come through.

For example, I've told you elsewhere to divide the human body into four quadrants.[5] The way we're built limits how many of these a person can protect at a time. The best of fighters can only cover three of these at one time, and "windows" only last a second. However, generally speaking most people can only cover two at once. That means the guy has two open windows for your attack to come through.

While this is true, I have to tell you that it's a generalization. When you get to the point where you're aiming for the fish's eye, if that guy is one side or the other off the quadrant's centerline, he's left an opening in that quadrant for you to come through. When my buddy Richard and I spar, we snake through holes in the other's defenses that are about 6 inches square! And that's me as a tired old fart! The more adept you become at this sort of thinking, the closer you come to the point where you won't look at someone and try to decide *if* you could take him out, you'll look at someone and know *how* you'd take him out.

Now that I've hopefully impressed on you the need for aiming at the fish's eye at all times, let's move on to battin' 'em onna da head. In many ways, force is like water or electricity. It will take the easiest path. That is, if it meets resistance it will either alter its course, blow through the resistance, or, if the resistance is big enough, come to a dead halt (after delivering all of its energy to whatever stopped it or bounce off after delivering a majority of its force).

Understand these four options, because one way or the other, they are exactly what you're going to do to rearrange someone's face. Now the first thing you need to realize is that the end ones are the ones that are really friendly to your moving. I mean, hey, you went through all the hassle

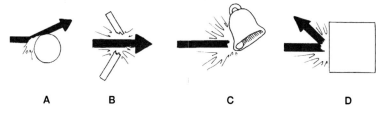

| A | B | C | D |

Figure 5. The four force options.

of letting gravity get you moving, so why stop it? Come to think of it, since we're going to talk about them a whole lot in this book, let's just name them now:

Option A: Redirecting force.
Option B: Splat! Blowing through.
Option C: Kaboom! Force delivered and stopped.
Option D: Ricochet. Not real original, but it's a new day and I haven't had my coffee yet so cut me some slack.

Look at the first option. This is what you want to do with your fall. When you first bunny hopped, your leg caught you and you hopefully stopped before you ran into anything. In scientific terms, your leg served as the instrument of Option C. While that is real nice to keep you from plowing into the coffee table, when it comes to delivering Nighty Nite Bunny Rabbits upside someone's head, you're going to want to use your leg as the instrument of Option A.

In other words, you don't want your leg to stop your motion, you want it to serve as the means to redirect it. Your pivoting creates the alternative direction your momentum is going to take, as shown in Figure 6.

This is the basic concept behind getting some serious oomph in your blows. Notice that the majority of the force is flowing along a curve.

To add extra energy, there are several things you can do. Start out by stomping your front foot when it lands. There are reasons for this, but I won't bore you with them. Secondly, drop your shoulder into the blow. This brings extra torque into your strike. The third thing is to

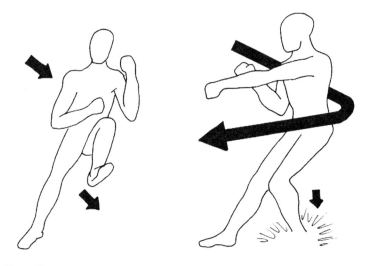

Figure 6.

keep your elbow, wrist, and shoulder tight. This itself serves three purposes: one, it transfers the entire force from your body mass through your arm and into your target. Two, by keeping everything tight it prevents your arm from turning into a shock absorber, which will decrease your blow's effectiveness. If things are all loosey goosey when you move, all the energy will not get delivered. What's the use of throwing a monster blow if half of it is going to be pissed off into the wind? And three, it keeps you from busting your hand or wrist from the impact. Useful, that. Oh yeah, and don't forget the centerline pivot.

All in all, though, the main whammy here comes from a simple thing called timing. Let me give you a great bit of fighting advice from a particularly weird source: cooking. One of the two key points that all cooking revolves around is getting everything to the table all at once and in the right condition. That means not only is everything ready to eat but when it gets there it's hot and not overcooked. In order to achieve this you gotta work on scheduling. Things that take longer to cook go on the stove first; things that cook fast (and cool just as fast) wait until the very last before starting.

If you've ever suffered through a meal from someone who didn't have this particular aspect of cooking down, you know how disastrous it can be. In the same vein, if you've ever taken a punch from someone who didn't have timing down, you probably didn't suffer any damage. That kind of defeats the purpose of a punch, doesn't it? Well bully for him for not having his shit together, but that ain't the way it's done around here, now is it?

Okay, take these factors and guess how much impact they'd muster:

1) Your entire body weight moving at about 20 miles an hour.
2) All of your strength.
3) Extra torque and speed brought about by a few more

minor motions. (35 mph? Ooooh, sounds painful. If you got it down, though . . .)

4) No shock absorbers or energy bleed through excess or wasted motion.
5) Being delivered through a hard part of your body.
6) Landing in an area that is extremely tender and vulnerable.
7) All of this being focused and delivered at the same moment.

It doesn't take an Einstein to realize that it would not be fun to be on the receiving end of a punch thrown by someone who's gotten all of these down. Them's all the component parts of a seriously nasty blow. If you ever feel that your blows either don't have any juice or aren't having any effect, I'll lay dollars to donuts that you're not doing one or more of those seven points.

If you haven't figured it out yet, your stomp/step needs to land at the same time that your punch lands. Why? Because the energy transference is that quick. You want all of your redirected energy to land on him. So, for a punch you want Option A to be happening on your side of the fence, but on his side you want all of your force to be doing an Option C into his ass. Ka-fucking-boom! Owww!

So in a nutshell, when you land one of these drop-step punches, start with your drop and spring off with your trailing foot. As you're falling, pivot (from the hips), pick your target, drop your shoulder (either down, in, or a combination, depending on where you're striking), throw your punch, ass in some muscle to add force and tighten your joints down, and culminate all action at the same moment that your foot slams onto the ground. It's now all come to the table at the right time and in the right condition.

Okay, one thing I hear a whole lot is people who say that they really can't learn how to do a move out of a book. Well, I have to agree with that. Honestly, you can't. The only way to learn something is to go out and practice it. You have to

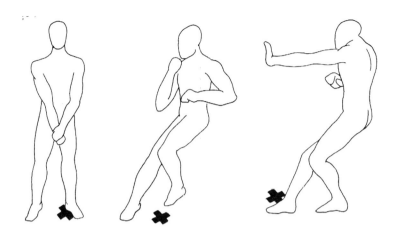

Figure 7. Falling punch.

know how it *feels* when it's done right. Your body is great for remembering how certain actions feel. It's part of a thing called kinetics.

Our bodies react to stay alive faster than we can consciously think to do so,[6] and there's a deep level in your body where such knowledge is imprinted. Generally, there are two ways to imprint this knowledge on this level, and both are based on experience. One is having actually been in a pretty hairy situation and found this level accidentally. You do what you gotta do to survive. The other thing is to practice, practice, practice until your body knows how to move this way. Then if you end up in a hairy situation, you will know how to react already. Guess which one you bleed less with. That's why practice is so important.

Even if you don't go out and study this stuff for 20 years, at least go out and devote a solid week to moving this way. Even if you don't ever practice it again, if you get into a shitstorm, your body will remember about aiming for the fish's eye and it will improve your chances of hitting it.

Now one of the things that really fucks up learning kinetics is your mind. Funny that your mind can interfere with your learning something, but it's true. There is a counter you can do to both keep that little monkey busy while you're trying to learn the kinetics and to learn faster. That is, put your mind to work analyzing where in the process you're losing energy (energy bleed, wasted motion, shock absorbers, loss of balance, etc.) and keep an eye on the timing. Did everything get to the table hot and all at once? If you find a problem with any of these issues, turn your logical mind loose on it. Everything not arriving at the same time? Figure out what needs to be started out earlier. Energy loss? Find where it's going. Loose shoulder? How about the pivot not being as tight as it could be. Any of these could lead to energy loss. Analyze, analyze, analyze!

Basically, what I just told you is exactly what your martial arts instructor is looking for when he stands there watching you before he corrects what you're doing. By turning your mind loose in this manner, you can learn it all a whole lot faster and better than if you just try to do it by rote memorization. It's really much easier than they make it out to be.

By the by, I highly recommend you read *Championship Fighting* by Jack Dempsey[7] for a much more detailed breakdown of this process. I definitely wouldn't want to have been hit by him. It's normally available in martial arts stores or in used bookstores under the same subject, or perhaps sports. (Also, if you're the sort who collects martial arts books, I recommend hitting used bookstores for your habit. They're cheaper there, and most of them end up there anyway.)

In case you haven't noticed it yet, I've just given you the tools you'll need to deliver one hell of a serious AI. I'm talking you're seriously going to be able to ring this guy's chimes. This simple first move is what will allow you to step in and do the first of several forthcoming AIs.

I'll tell you, the only thing more demoralizing to him than his attack failing to even connect is realizing he's just received a punch that is more powerful than anything he could throw. Not only will he be dealing with the shock of everything suddenly going wrong and getting his bells tolled, but he also might realize that he's stepped into the ring with a Tasmanian devil who's got a whole lot more in store for him. While he's trying to figure out what the hell went wrong, though, you're already on the way to ending the whole thing right quick. That bone-rattling thwack you just gave him is only the beginning . . .

Remember: the effectiveness of even the most powerful blow is lessened if it doesn't hit in a tender spot, while the effectiveness of the same blow in a vital spot is tenfold!

Here are some of my favorite choice targets for impact AIs:

Back of the jaw, near the ear
Side of the neck
Collarbone
Short ribs
Diaphragm
Kidneys
Groin

Connecting with any one of these will get his attention. Hitting three or four will definitely take the fight out of anyone short of a maniac/PCP freakout. Again, as a blatant and mercenary plug . . . er, I mean, as a vital source of information, I recommend you read *Fists, Wits, and a Wicked Right* for more details about nonimpact AIs.

ENDNOTES

1. There are three common kinds of blows. The setup is for getting your opponent to expose the real target you're after. These blows are done fast, without much body weight, and cause little actual damage. Rattlers rattle your opponent. They're heavier punches, usually slower, and cause cumulative damage. Nighty Nite Bunny Rabbits are the heavy punches that end the fight. These blows are explained in detail in my first book, *Cheap Shots, Ambushes, and Other Lessons.*

Gettin' a Move On

2. Like in damn near everything I've ever written.

3. Occasionally *one* well-placed hard blow is more effective than ten of the same, but by using two or three you work closer to a guaranteed "more effective."

4. From *Tactics of Mistake* by Gordon R. Dickson, part of the Dorsai Series. By the way, I highly recommend this sci-fi series. It's about a planet of mercenaries and how they evolve into supersoldiers.

5. Matter of fact, if you look in Appendix E you can get a quick rundown.

6. Which leads to a thing called the Tichner response, which is an autonomic reaction to certain stimuli.

7. For those of you of tender years (i.e., under 70), Jack Dempsey was the heavyweight boxing champion from 1919 to 1926. He wrote the book in 1950.

CHAPTER 5

Counters, Blocks, Czechs, and Even a Pole

Incoming fire has the right of way.
—Murphy's Law of Combat #18

While you're in the process of moving toward the annihilation of the shmuck who has attacked you, you may want to consider the feasibility of deflecting or warding off any attack that he may have instigated. Admit it, it looks better if you don't have to go to the hospital with the guy you just put there.

Fortunately this can usually be done much easier now that you're no longer standing where you were a moment ago. Now I want you to notice something here. Take a look at Figure 8.

Much blood can be saved by understanding this simple little illustration. Keep it in mind as I meander around the subject for a while. We will get back to it again and again and again.

One thing that I've pissed and moaned about (other than my phone bill) is how the martial arts apparently have the concept of defense ass backwards. Their primary line of defense is also their first, if not only, line of defense. This might work in the dojo or tournament, but it's suicide out in the real world. Why? Because of Murphy! If Murphy wasn't lurking around the corner, this might work, but he's out there

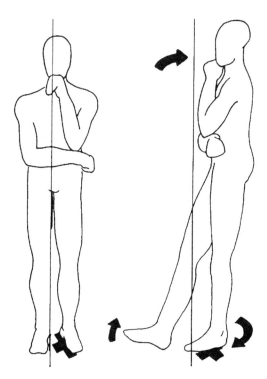

Figure 8. Body pivot.

waiting to come crash the party! "Martial arts perspective, meet Murphy. Murphy, martial arts perspective. Have fun."

From what it looks like to the newcomer, martial artists are putting their entire safety on the strength of their blocks alone. That's it! One line of defense! Man, your reality check just bounced. If that block does not successfully stop an attack, you're screwed! Of course this will be fervently denied by most martial artists, but waiting six months or more before focusing on something as basic as stepping off the line of attack kinda indicates scrambled priorities to me.[1] All talk about discipline and having to know how to punch, block, and kick aside, if someone wants to know how not to get hurt by a mugger, it makes more sense to me to give him something that works right now. However, my idea of what the "basics" are tend to be a little different than most. But then, having survived a couple dances with drunks, gang-bangers, drug freakouts, knife- and club-wielding assholes, pissed-off husbands, et al, what do I know?

Now, if you're just dealing with a guy who's trying to punch you, maybe just a single block will work. It happens . . . occasionally, especially because most people don't know how to punch worth a damn. Most "powerful" punches are usually slow, obvious, and relatively easy to block, while the fast ones seldom carry the clout they need to really hurt you. In these sorts of situations, having the attitude that your blocks will do everything for you is fine. They keep out the heavy blows, and the lighter ones are just sucked up. Personally, though, I think this is an attitude for tournament fighters, would-be supermen, and people who've never had someone actually try to kill them.

However, by now you've realized that A) anytime you engage in violence there are no limits on how far it can and will go, and B) anytime it could end up with you or him dead, it sort of changes what you think about the whole sheebang. This awareness can either come about from personal or professional experience and is best summed up in the sage saying, "shit happens."

What really amazes me is the number of people who insist that the only way to be safe against an attack is to do something counterinstinctive. That means train yourself to automatically do something other than what seems to be the smart move at the time (i.e., duck when someone tries to punch your lights out). The prevailing attitude in many places is if something comes at you, you have to counterattack and overwhelm it. He attacks, you blow his attack out of the water, then charge in! Grrr! Me heap big grizzly bear! Me no fear nothing! Me tear him new asshole! (A foot on your dead opponent and beating on your chest while doing a Tarzan yell afterwards is optional.) Gosh, that's exactly what I want to do . . . NOT!

Counters, Blocks, Czechs and Even a Pole

If I may use computer terms here for a moment, I will explain much of the problem that people have learning what these yahoos are calling self-defense.[2] Understanding this will not only help you now, but it will also help you when you go out and start teaching. (What? You think you can get by without passing on the torch? HA!!!!)

Basically, what I call self-defense training is supposed to instill in you a new set of tools to handle an extreme and difficult situation. When it comes to tools, what works best are automatic reflexes—those things you do instinctively when you receive certain cues or stimuli. Supposedly, this new self-defense system trains and shapes what you will do instinctively to protect yourself.

However, as you're standing here right now, you have certain tools and applications already running. Came with the package, it did. Where most people have problems learning self-defense is that instead of just doing the smart thing and writing an extension onto the person's pre-existing program, most martial arts instructors are trying to install an entirely new contradictory system. This new system works fine for them in their hardware but is totally foreign to their students. Mr. Martial Artist is on a different computer than you are! After years of training, what he does instinctively is not what you do instinctively. It's like trying to run Macintosh software on an IBM.

At best, this leads to system collision—two programs that are not compatible slamming into each other and neither one working. If you've ever felt like a klutz in a martial arts class, you know what I'm talking about. It just don't work for where you are right now! Why? Because even if you do manage to run that program, it is not instinctive to you. It's not how you would normally react until you have lots and lots more experience.

While counterattacking is an option, it's not your normal reaction—that is, unless you've spent years of normal training or months of intensive training. What is your normal reaction to someone throwing a brick at your head?

Do you stand there and try to catch it? Do you just contemptuously slap it aside while glowering at the guy who threw it? FUCK NO! You duck and try to slap it away! That is what you do instinctively! Wanna know something? *What you do instinctively is what you do faster!*

Unless you have been thoroughly brainwashed or have balls the size of Cincinnati, your first reaction is going to be to flinch away. Maybe a split second later you'll say "fuck this" and attack, but A precedes B with nearly everyone. If you try and change the process and put B out there as your first reaction, one of two things will occur:

1) Four things will simultaneously collide at high speed: system A, system B, his fist, and your face.
2) You will be a graduate of the United States Marine Corps boot camp.

Neither of those options are real conducive to being around in good shape to lie to your grandkids.[3] In all honesty, your best chance is to take what you got now and write an extension program that makes it work more effectively. If your natural instinct is to flinch away from an attack, then do it! And don't feel bad about it! With a little tweaking it can be more effective than you can possibly dream. And 99 times out of 100 it's more effective than standing there like a stud muffin and trying to block the attack.

I've met a lot of people who are uncomfortable because their first reaction to violence isn't to immediately knock bullets out of the air with their dicks. People often mistake brainwashing and testosterone for fighting skill. Believe me, they are not the same. Unless you are a professional sports fighter or in the military, it's not about winning the fight, it's about surviving the best you can. In this case, by ending it quickly, you increase your chances of surviving unscathed. Forget what the butch thing to do is, you do what works best for you, because if you've tweaked it a little, it will work just fine.

Counters, Blocks, Czechs and Even a Pole

Now generally speaking, if you are successful at your first reaction of flinching away from an attack, your next reaction will be either fear or anger. It has been my experience that the more successful you are at avoiding the attack, the more likely you are to get pissed. Which is not a bad thing. If his attack missed you by a hair or, just as importantly, you feel it did, the odds are you are going to be more scared than pissed. While concern is a good thing, fear isn't. Fear can get in the way and make you panic and/or freeze. This is why you need to practice getting out of the way (it's called slipping, by the way). That way you know the dude missing wasn't a fluke but directly related to what you did! The more experience you have slipping and checking, the less scary attacks become.

This is why if you don't practice anything else in this book, you should do the following exercise. For at least a week just practice slipping. You and a partner go out and start slow. He throws single punches at you. Don't do anything but practice doing the drop step to the side and pivoting. (Well okay, you can learn to watch his shoulders for the subtle body cues of a punch being prepared to be thrown if you want to.) It might make it easier if you hold your hands behind your back while doing this. During this time you're not really trying to hit each other. It's just to get you into the habit of slipping. Start slow and pick up speed. Still no hands yet.

Once you've gotten to the point where you've got the hang of the motion and have picked up speed, it's time to add in the checks. Practice, practice, practice! Still do not try to really hit each other. Do this until you've gotten to the point where you can calmly face a pretend punch and slip/check it out of the way. Then pick up speed. Once you've gotten to the point where you can calmly slip a fast pretend punch, then it is time for the next level.

If you're smart you'll wear boxing gloves from here on in. If you want to learn much faster but at a higher risk to yourself, do this bare-handed. I personally recommend the gloves and mouthguards for beginners, but you do what you want to do. (If you get a broken nose or lose a tooth, don't blame me!) Now, starting with light blows, really try to hit each other. (You're still throwing single shots.) Again, practice the slipping and checking until you've got it down. Up the level to whatever you're comfortable with.

Now comes the graduation. Still doing the single shots, throw a punch in anger. Inside your head get mean, get vicious, get angry, and throw a punch that you intend to land. You are trying to hurt the fucker with your punch. It's up to the slipper to avoid it. When you throw a punch you are also throwing anger. Swap off. Do this for a while until you can avoid any kind of blow thrown at you. Then amp down and go back to practicing regular pulled punches.

This does several things, most of them out on a woo-woo sounding level, but they are issues of critical importance. Most important is that it slowly conditions you to calmly face someone's anger while they are attacking. Seldom are real punches thrown without anger. If you are not familiar with facing this energy, no matter how much you've trained in a dojo (where punches are thrown calmly and nonviolently), you're going to hesitate when you meet up with the real thing—the screaming, angry, out-of-control guy who's sincerely dedicated to busting your jaw! Putting it in esoteric terms, you're facing the guy's chi as well as his attack. Those two things together are what scares most people. By training with them you lessen the terror they hold.

If you have successful experience dealing with both anger and attacks, when you meet up with that particular combination in the street you'll know how to handle it and be able to react in time. While you may say "oh shit," you won't go "EEEEEEK!" and freeze up. This is what defeats most people who have trained for self-defense: while they trained to handle the physical moves, they didn't train to handle the energy that they will be dealing with too. Incidentally, the ability to go "oh shit (slip), I gotta end this

fast (kaboom)" is often mistaken for THONGOR COUN-
TERATTACK (as in Thongor the Learning Impaired). But
one is using your head while the other is the result of either
brainwashing or testosterone poisoning. You figure out
which is which.

I cannot begin to tell you how many people have told me
that they cannot dodge that fast. Sometimes they're too big,
too fat, their reactions aren't fast enough, etc., etc. Man, if
you can walk, you can do this! The same motion that carries you over to blow someone into next week is the one
that will get your ass out of the way. Face it, while it is better
to be able to move fast, you're not just relying on moving to
save you. You can block on top of all of this. When you add
in a slew of blocks, counters, checks, and kitchen sinks, you
will slow him down. Even if your block isn't totally effective, by the time his attack gets through, even a tortoise
could have managed to get out of the way.

Believe it or not, just by slipping you've done about
three things to put your opponent's dick in the mud.
Number one, you've avoided his attack. Unless he's really
well trained, it comes as a major "huh?" surprise to most
people when they throw a punch and it misses entirely.
He's expecting his fist to hit your face and is often thrown
off his stride when the expected is replaced by the unexpected. This gives you a mental edge. Number two, it sort of
follows that most people who are surprised by the first
issue didn't figure on the resistance of your face not being
there. In fact, most of them were expecting to use your face
to stop their forward motion. This unexpected lack of
resistance often throws them off balance. Oddly enough,
there are entire fighting systems designed around the guy
making this kind of error. Number three is you've moved
off his primary line of orientation. Generally, that too causes a skip in most people's CD while they try and figure out
exactly what the hell happened.

Note Figure 9. The first illustration shows how most
people are oriented. Front, back, side to side. Pretty simple.

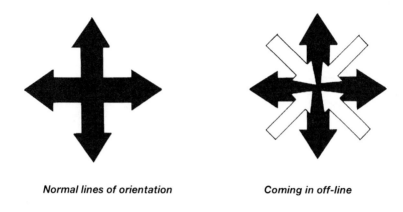

Normal lines of orientation   *Coming in off-line*

Figure 9. Lines of orientation.

Now odds are that laughing boy had you targeted in his forward orientation. You're in front of him; he's punching you. That's front orientation. Not real sophisticated but often real effective. However when something slips off the cleanly defined 90 degree lines of orientation (as shown in the second illustration), it confuses a lot of people. The first reaction of most people is to stop, pull back, and reorient, then launch another attack (Figure 10).

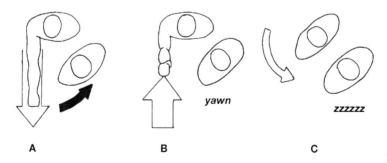

A   B   C

Figure 10. Reorientating after a slipped attack. Illustration A shows the attack and the slip. In B, the attacker pulls back his attack. In C, he shifts position, again oriented on the front line.

Counters, Blocks, Czechs and Even a Pole

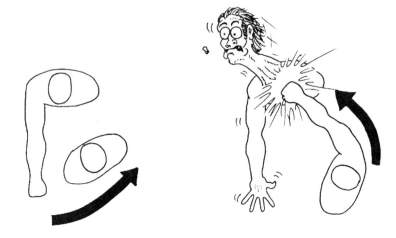

Figure 11.

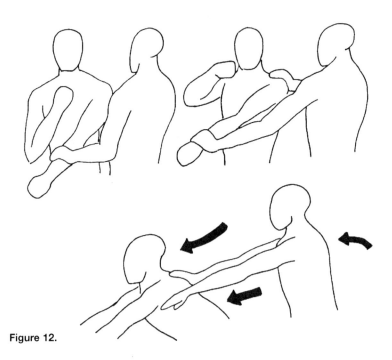

Figure 12.

A Professional's Guide to Ending Violence Quickly

That's normal and that's what you want him to do. Because while bozo is taking all that time to go through his dog-and-pony show, you're going to show him that there are people who simultaneously attack while they reorient themselves, like in Figure 11.

The fourth thing you've done by slipping is put the guy in a situation where he's got to crawl all over himself to get another clear shot at you. In other words, you've crossed him up. From this position he has to either spend all sorts of time doing the stop/draw back/reorient (time he doesn't have) or try to take a shot at you over himself (difficult, unwieldy, lacking in power, and not real effective). This is the normal reaction. See Figure 12.

Now FYI, there are a few ways out of this sort of situation. I'll tell you them for two reasons: 1) So you can practice them, thereby making the counters I'm going to talk about less effective if some tacky shmuck has the audacity to try the same on you. Remember, your best and nastiest move should work on someone else, not on you. 2) In case you have the bad luck to cross a trained fighter who knows how to counter your check. When you feel him countering your move, *immediately* stop what you are doing and shift to some other move.

While both are important for keeping your face intact, I have real strong feelings about number 2. I cannot tell you how many people out there are trained in what I consider a suicidal manner. Once they start a move, they intend to finish it no matter what else is going on around them. Now I want you to realize that a major part of what I'm going to mention in this chapter is reliant on some fool thinking this way. An important safety tip is, if you're going to curl your lip in disdain at someone, it is considered wise if you don't turn around and do the same thing that you're sneering at him for doing.

Probably the best and fastest way out of many of the things I'm going to describe is to simply drop your elbow. If you're winging out a vertical punch, you can just drop it straight down. If you're throwing a regular (horizontal) punch, you'll need to roll your arm so your elbow is pointed down before you drop it (Figure 13).

Hopefully you'll catch on that I broke the second one into two parts for clarification, not as how you have to do it. In other words, you can both spin and drop at once. Once you've slipped out of it, do one of them reorientation/shift/counterattack all-rolled-into-one moves that we've been talking about (Figure 14). Another way to handle this situation is, if the guy has landed his check on your forearm instead of your elbow, just fold your arm back. What he's pushing on suddenly evaporates. If he's trained, he'll stop pushing and start protecting against your forthcoming attack (all in all an ugly situation, but better than what would have happened). If he's not, his arm goes flying by, exposing his entire side and neck. This leaves you in the perfect position to backfist the sucker or come in with a pivot-backed sucker punch (Figure 15).

Even if you don't get to shift his nose after folding your arm, your elbow is out there to hold him off and keep him from stepping in with a real serious uppercut. Since you're going to be rolling away from the situation anyway, this should be enough. (You *are* going to be rolling away from the situation, by the way, right?)

A more advanced counter is to do the elbow drop with a countercheck. At this point I should warn you that you're heading in "two snakes fucking" territory, commonly referred to as "infighting." Most of the moves that I've mentioned have been "yipee kiyay wide open range" sort of stuff in comparison to where this kind of move leads to. Infighting is a type of fighting where everything is done at point-blank range and the moves are so fast, subtle, and convoluted that one three-second engagement can have as many as eight different moves from each side. Counters, checks, and blocks fly by at incredible speed. I've had trained martial artists lose the chain of events of a sparring match between Richard and I (he's the guy I did the knife

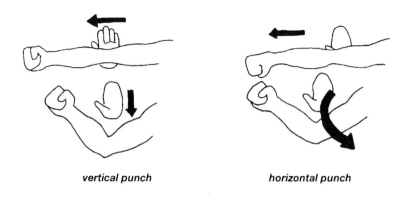

vertical punch   *horizontal punch*

Figure 13. Elbow drops.

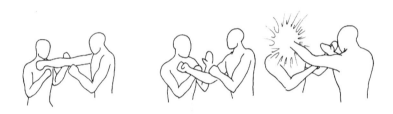

Figure 14. Elbow drop/counterattack.

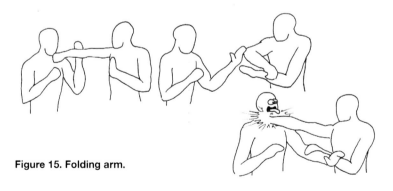

Figure 15. Folding arm.

Counters, Blocks, Czechs and Even a Pole

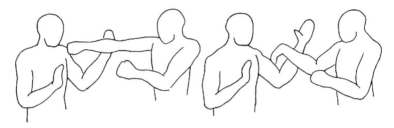
Figure 16. Elbow drop/countercheck.

video with, by the way) after the first second. We step back and ask, "How many times you get hit?" The guy with the lower score wins that round. Sort of like wolverines playing a twisted version of golf. If you're interested in this sort of nastiness, go out and study kali, escrima, arnis, pentjak silat, and snake porno films.

Now that I've shown you how to mess up what you're going to learn, let's get onto the fine points of the business. First things first: what's the difference between a check and a counter and a block?

Here, let's make it easy. Look at Figure 17.

You may have noticed that there are four illustrations for three options. That's because there is one choice that is repeated twice. A counter can be either A or D. Sorry about any confusion this may cause, but it's a limitation of the English language. Unless I wanted to use some sort of mouth-fulla-marbles term from a remote place that

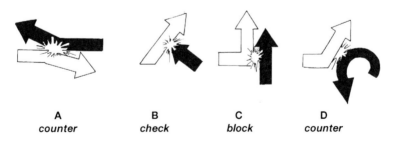

| A | B | C | D |
| counter | check | block | counter |

Figure 17.

A Professional's Guide to Ending Violence Quickly

nobody has ever heard of, we're stuck with the same word describing two related actions. Generally you just gotta learn contextual usage to know which one someone is talking about. For clarification's sake, however, I'll refer to them as Counter A and Counter D

Since we're talking about them already, let's address counters first. A counter is a force which is applied to an incoming force that deflects the incoming force. Now it can be an outgoing force moving along basically a parallel line (as in Counter A) that derails the incoming force while delivering a rude surprise to the attacker (that's why it's called a counterpunch). This kind of move takes a lot of practice to perfect, but it is an absolute mother to defend against. You have to be on your toes and really be able to read your opponent's body language to make this work. You have to see him prepare to throw a blow and instantly fire off the counterstrike. Your blow hits his and you snake in on the inside. Or if you've remembered to slip his attack, you can come up along his outside, which is better because it also crosses him up.

A counter can also be a deflecting force applied to the incoming force that blows it off line. By itself such an action works best the closer it is applied to the incoming force's source of origin, but it can also be combined with blocks and the first type of counter for truly spectacular effects. Believe it or not, the most common counter is simply a rotation of the wrist. If you can flip your hand from palm up to palm down (as in Figure 18), you can do a counter.

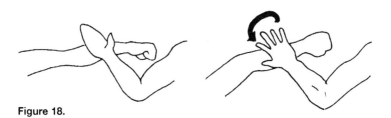

Figure 18.

Counters, Blocks, Czechs and Even a Pole

Go out and try this experiment. Have someone hold out their relaxed arm toward you. Then place your hand flat on his biceps. Now, keeping your hand in basically the same place, quickly rotate your palm. (If you can't find a partner, use an open door.) Use your middle finger as the pivot point—it stays in the same place while your hand and forearm spin. As you get the hang of this, extend that imaginary line running down your finger out through your hand, wrist, and, eventually, forearm. After a while, when you spin, it's your entire forearm that's supplying power to your counter, not just your palm. Believe it or not, this little refinement can turn this move into a real powerhouse.

If the person's arm was pointed at your chest, this simple action should deflect his arm at least out to your shoulder or thereabouts. Don't worry if it doesn't, though; it can take some practice. Also, I've only given you half of the system thus far, and your opponent isn't moving, which has a lot to do with it.

What I want you to try now is do the same pivot on a person's extended arm, but this time do it at their wrist. While it still does have an effect, it shouldn't have moved it more to about the middle of either of your pectoral muscles. While this and a jerk of your head can save you from a fist in the face, the farther from the guy's shoulder (the blow's point of origin) you do it, the less effective it is. Not useless, just less effective.

Counter D is a real mother to deal with when it is combined with any of the other three options. There are all sorts of reasons why this small, subtle move can increase the efficiency of nearly every move you can do (punches, blocks, counters, et al), but if you want a mind-grinding explanation for why, go tackle a physics major and have him explain it. All you need to know is that anything you do can be supercharged by simply adding in this simple rotation of the forearm. It's called torque.

Instead of just punching straight, a rotation of your forearm adds in extra torque, which means a harder hit.

Anyone who's ever been hit by an experienced fighter can tell you their blows hurt more. Well, this is one of the reasons why. The combination of mass, torque, and body weight being delivered all at once can knock someone into next week.

A check can be delivered from only 3 inches away, and by adding that flick of the wrist at first contact, this subtle move can have the same devastating strength of a full-on block and blow your opponent's arm as much as 2 feet off course. All from a movement that takes up no more than 6 inches. However a full-on check aided by this wrist pivot at the second of impact and where you follow through with the check can take the guy to where he's hopping around trying to keep from falling over on his face. And he ain't going to be able to muster a good counterattack from that position.

The hardest blow most people can muster can be easily deflected by adding this wrist pivot into your blocks. If you still want to stand there and slug it out with the dude, seriously incorporate this little wrist spin into your blocks, as it increases their effectiveness tenfold.

The trick to these moves comes in two parts. Number one is, it is easier to affect mass in motion than it is to affect it when it's stationary. With one you're using its own energy against it, while with the other you're doing all the work. Putting it simply, it's easier to derail a moving train than it is to push a standing one over. That's because you're not trying to take total control of their mass and energy; all you're doing is taking away *their* control of those two factors, which will cause them to crash and burn. Remember, by slipping you've left the dude rolling ahead with no brakes, and at that moment he is real susceptible to being derailed. This makes him vulnerable to small, intense applications of force.

The second part of the trick is timing. This twist has to happen (or be at its height) when you contact with the incoming force. You do not connect and then begin to

Counters, Blocks, Czechs and Even a Pole

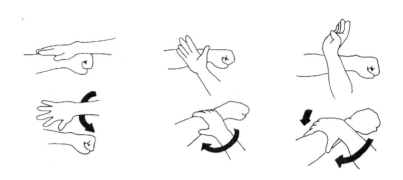

Figure 19.

twist; you're torquing *as* you contact. This means you're hitting him with two forces in combination. You start your move and at the last second throw in the twist. When you make contact, both of them are in full swing (Figure 19).

A check deflects his force by either spinning him in a different direction or causing him to trip up by throwing counterenergy into what he is doing. In either case, the guy will end up being either crossed up or blown aside. Most commonly, checks are delivered with the flat of your hand. Now depending on how you do them, they can either be done with just your arm or all of your body weight.

Your opponent's attack is deflected away from you. Much of the reaction comes from how much juice he put into his punch and how much he was relying on your snot

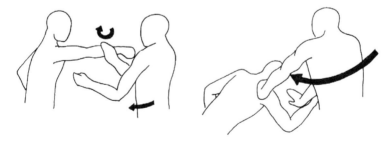

Figure 20. The check.

A Professional's Guide to Ending Violence Quickly

locker to serve as his brakes. The harder the guy is throwing an off-balanced punch and the more he was looking for you to supply his safety net, the more off-kilter he is when you check him. Naturally, if you happened to include some of your body weight from the step/pivot and extra energy from a slap block or wrist pivot, this would be a whole lot more effective no matter what he was doing right or wrong.

The second one you'll notice has all sorts of interesting things going on. What is most important to realize is that the kind of check I'm applying here has my entire body weight behind it. It's not a matter of his fist hitting my body weight; it's my weight hitting his arm and consequently him. How my weight is being delivered is through my checking hand. Now I don't care how strong someone is, nobody can handle 160 pounds slamming into their arm!

Either of these particular moves tends to put your opponent in an awkward position. The less trained or more drunk he is, the more this is really going to mess him up. Generally, it puts him in a position where it is incredibly easy to take him down. I'm talking three quarters of the work is done for you already, and all you need to do is give a little shove or pull or extend a foot and gravity and his own inertia will do the rest. Of course, the AI you lay on him as he's going past you on the way to the ground doesn't hurt either. In the absolute best-case scenario, a check will cause someone to fall over all by himself. In the worst case, all it did was keep you from getting punched or stabbed. Don't that sound just awful?

Now the number one thing to know about checks is that they really, really are dependent on you being able to aim for the fish's eye. The best, most effective checks are done on the guy's elbow. The reasons are nearly endless. From there you can spin his entire body around by just pivoting or stepping forward. You can follow any move or counter he may attempt, making it useless. Most people don't realize the vulnerability of the elbow or the danger, so they don't react as fast as they would against a recognizable attack. People are prone to try to resist with muscles instead of doing the smart thing and rolling away. This makes them more susceptible to any pressure you apply. You can predict anything the guy is going to try to do to escape or attack and simply move to a place where it won't be effective. This is why experienced fighters say, "He who controls the elbow controls the fight."

I want you to try something with your sparring partner. Go out one day and just put your hand on his elbow and no matter what he does, just follow it. Step up, step back, twist, turn, extend your arm, retract your arm. Just stay to the guy's side and play with it. Now with your hand still on his elbow, have him try and hit you with that hand. Just block and push him away.

When you do that, it may come as a surprise to you the direct correlation between you losing contact with his elbow and the times you got hit. There are more than a few reasons why a check is good for not getting hit.

Obviously the last option is the block. I've ranted and raved about blocks elsewhere and many a time. Generally, I have found these other two options to be faster and more effective, but there are times when a block is just the thing to have around. My recommendation is that you go out and learn the slap/whip blocks I've described and that are shown in my videos and books, because they are really just as nasty and effective as what I've been talking about here.

ENDNOTES

1. But hey, that's why I'm considered a barbarian. That and tacky comments like, "I understand the concept of dying for tradition, but shouldn't that choice be made by the person doing the dying?" Hoooh, that one went over well with the martial arts world, let me tell you!

2. Here's a philosophical chew toy for you of the IQ set. I divide the "martial arts" into four distinct categories: 1) self-defense, 2) a physical art/discipline, 3) a spiritual path, and 4) a sport. Each has

its own focus, intent, and training that really isn't useful outside its own field of specialty. The question is, why do I say that the average 39th degree danny has probably not mastered more than two of these at most? I've met 80-year-old grandmasters who freely admit that they've only mastered three aspects. If you want to argue with me about this, you can reach me via e-mail at AnimalMac@aol.com.

3. Nothing personal guys. It's just when it comes to war, I prefer Sun Tzu's strategy over Brier Bear's, "Les jes bash 'im onna head." While a hammer is a useful tool, a well-stocked tool chest looks mighty appealing to a tired old fart like me.

CHAPTER 6

Awwwwww!
He Fell Down!
(Okay So He Had a Little Help)

"I could hit him with my hand, or I could hit him with the earth. The earth is much bigger and it hurts more to be hit with it."

—Pendakar

I cannot begin to stress enough how important it is to get your opponent down to the ground as soon as possible. Remember, the goal is to end the violence ASAP. You may have to add to his distress with one or two Attitude Interrupters before you take him down, but in all honesty you should try to avoid doing more than three moves before you introduce him to Mother Earth. The sooner that guy hits the ground, the less likely he is to get a piece out of you.

Collectively, the combination of AIs and him hitting the ground is really going to put a dent in his style. A guy down on the ground isn't much of a threat to you. Even if he has a gun, that trip to the ground is going to distract him big time while you hot foot it away!

Besides, have you ever taken a serious header? How fast did you want to do anything other than lay there and hope the pain went away? "Nah man, I jes wanna lay here and groan for awhile, thank you very much." How fast he's going to find his marbles depends on how hard you chose to slam the asshole. There's a reason pro football players lay there for a second after a tackle. Even with all the protective gear they wear, they've often just gotten their bells rung by slamming into the ground. The harder the hit, the longer they lay there!

Now, just as there are thousands of ways to deliver a blow, there are thousands of ways to get someone down on the ground. Sound complicated? It's not. Every way of getting the guy to the ground consists of one thing. *Gravity*. Nothing more—one way or the other, putting the guy in a situation where he follows gravity. Whether this is throwing him, tripping him, knocking him over, or giving him a choice between a broken arm or hurling himself onto the ground, it doesn't matter. Him going to the ground is him following gravity!

There are three ways to achieve this glorified state:

1) Take his balance away.
2) Take his support away
3) Put him into a situation where he is "slaved" to your motion.

Every technique you will ever come across is based on one or more of these fundamentals. Try to think of one that isn't. I've got more than 25 years experience with the fine arts of murder, mayhem, destruction, and despair, and I can't think of one that isn't covered by these three. Even the most obscure wrist lock you can find is based on slaving him to your body's motion (i.e., he follows you or gets a broken something or other). You lock him up (slave him) and then what happens? You force him to move some way so he loses his balance and gravity takes over. Or if you want to get real traditional, you go down too! Maybe not as far as him, but you follow gravity and he not only comes with but goes farther than you.

A quick summation of these three principles looks something like this. The throwing techniques, dragging him over, and just plain tackling the fucker are examples of taking his balance away (number 1). Tripping, leg sweeps, and blowing out his kneecaps take his support away (number 2). Grabbing something tender and/or locking his joints just before you apply your downward-moving body weight is slaving him to your motion (number 3). Did I miss any options? I don't think so. Some of the nastiest moves are really cool combinations of all of the above.

Take a branding iron and burn these three fundamentals into your brain. From now on, every time you learn a new technique, figure out which file it belongs in and stick it there. Not only will it help you learn faster, but your understanding of the underlying principles that make all of this tick will allow you to wing it when a "proper" technique isn't possible.

In other words, you can make your own techniques to fit the situation—improvised techniques that are more effective than the proper/traditional technique would be under the circumstances. Now I may be speaking heresy from a traditionalist point of view ("That's not a proper technique!"), but I always figured my ass is more important than doing it the way some guy 500 years ago came up with. And if laughing boy could figure it out, so can I, and so can you. And I can tell you from personal experience, when it comes to violence, fuck the art, get the job done.

Moving right along, let us never forget that not only is gravity pressing against you but also against the asshole who is bracing you. That's what makes those three means of getting him to the ground so effective. If he loses his control over gravity, he will fall down just as fast as you do. I don't care how big he is, how bad he is, how well-trained he is, or even how freaked out on booze or drugs he is. Gravity affects everyone the same. It's an equal-opportunity force of nature.

Now I want to loop back to something here for a second. Want to hear the voice of experience? I'm talking on the street, in the bar, live-fire, "hey this kinda shit happens" experience. It's not something that happens in the dojo too often. It's also something that people who teach this sort of stuff often forget to mention, but here it is: *the guy ain't going to go to the ground willingly!* In fact, odds are if he ain't busy trying to wiggle his way out of it, he's trying to take your ass with him!

I wrote a book on floor fighting (called *Floor Fighting*, oddly enough), and in it I wrote about a thing called the "point of no return." This is the point in your balance where, I don't care who you are, unless you have wings you're going down. Hasta la vista, baby! You're going over. I also mentioned that the reason most people get hurt going to the ground is because they're still trying to get upright after they've passed the point of no return. In other words, instead of preparing for a landing, they're still trying to stay up. Hitting the ground is not only a shock but, believe it or not, *it's a surprise.* They didn't expect to fall over. Since they didn't expect it, they didn't prepare for it. Since they didn't prepare for it, they got hurt when it happened.

Now while what I just described is true for most people (especially drunks), there are two nasty exceptions, and these exceptions are real mothers to deal with. One is the trained fighter who not only knows what's happening and what to do about it, he's gonna intentionally mess up your move too, or, in a worse case, take your ass with him. If he's going, so are you! How he does it could be really tricky. You go to drop him by snagging up his legs, and he does the same to you. Or my personal fav, you grab and chuck him and he grabs on, possibly slamming a knee into your leg as he goes. Now you're slaved to *his* falling body weight with your support missing. EEEeeewwwgh!

The other way is when the guy who suddenly feels himself going over and just flails around trying to grab any support available. Since you're the closest thing that he can grab onto, guess who's going to be selected? Suddenly there's a kicking and screaming guy dangling off your shoulder, and if he's anywhere other than on your line of stance integrity, you've got some problems. This isn't training or skill, just Mr. Murphy and his damn law showing up.

Both situations end up with you going to the ground instead of just him. If you didn't catch on when reading *Floor Fighting*, the ground is where people are most likely to die in bare-handed conflicts. Going to the ground can very easily lead to you going *into* the ground. You can be stomped to death by the guy's friends real easy while down there. Someone can pick up a chair and swat you like a bug. You can slam into tables and chairs on the way down. You can fall on (and break) beer bottles, mugs, glasses, etc., or any other of a wide variety of ugly situations. All of which is why you really want to avoid going there in a real street conflict.

Don't rely on the kindness of strangers if you've just broken their buddy's arm and you're now lying on the ground. They will grind you like a cigarette butt. I've seen people stomped, beaten, chain whipped, and clubbed while they were down there, so don't think it couldn't happen to you.

Believe it or not, though, both scenarios where you go down with Chuckles can be prevented with what you learned in the counters and checks chapter. How? That same move that keeps you from getting your pretty face mushed up also keeps the guy from glomming onto your ass.

Here's a free bit of advice for any would-be Morihei Ueshibas: *Always expect the son of a bitch to try and take you down with him or, worse, slide something into your gut while he's going down!*

By being mentally prepared for the possibility, you automatically cover your butt, thereby lessening the chance of it happening. In fact, I always recommend you keep one hand ready to block any attempt on his part to either grab you or pop you one as he's going down. A wildly flung hand that grabs on can drag your ass down right quick. If the dude has a knife or razor, that wild hand is even uglier. This ain't the movies—you don't always see the weapon in the guy's hand. (Many a street fighter has been acquitted because at no time did anyone see any weapon. Everyone saw him punch the guy, but since nobody saw—or could later find— a blade, savvy lawyers got them off.) Granted the dude having a weapon is a worst-case scenario, but every year there are nearly half a million people who either die or are hospitalized because of this same "worst-case" scenario. Many of them are people who came to armed combat with the idea that it was going to be a fistfight.

Your best chance against surviving a weapon attack is in quicktime fighting. That fucker is trying to stab you! The only thing that will keep you from getting carved is if you quicktime him! No matter who you are, if you're out running where the wild things play, you'd better remember that there ain't no limits.

This particular bit of advice is another one of those little things that separate me from most martial arts instructors. I don't care about just putting an opponent on the floor. I'm more concerned with putting him down some way where he is not a threat anymore. And that includes *while* he's going down. Remember, in the dojo you ain't training with someone who's trying to resist you and hurt you. In the street that's exactly what will happen. I cannot tell you the number of times I've seen looks of shock on the faces of judo and aikido practitioners when I'd glommed onto them and we both went down. There I am in mid-flight with everything going hunky dory as far as he was concerned, and all of a sudden I twist like a cat and everything goes to hell in a handbasket.

So even though you may have the guy going down, remember that the threat still exists! You gotta guard against it or you can be victimized by it, whether intentionally or by dumb luck on the guy's part. You've just put into motion some serious physics (his body weight falling), so don't stop for a cigarette in the middle of the process. You wouldn't open a gate and let a mad bull loose into the same ring with you and just stop and hang out, now would you? It's the same thing. Until you get *all* the way to safety, don't chill out.

Perhaps the most important thing to realize about this is it's more a matter of attitude. Many people tend to mentally relax once a move starts to work. Once they think it's going fine, they sort of go on autopilot. But until the sucker bounces once or twice and shows obvious signs that he is not interested in continuing the aggression, you had better keep on your toes and make sure he doesn't take another shot at you!

Now I want to concentrate on the topic of taking someone's balance away. Not to be too terribly technical, but there are basically only two ways to do this: pushing and pulling. Either you push the guy off balance or you pull him off balance. Everything else is just details and how hard you want to work. Following my tendency to boil everything down to the basics and let you play with the details, I want you to take a peek at Figure 21.

Generally, the person who understands the concepts these illustrations convey is the person who is going to be still standing when the mess is over. And yes, the information is that simple . . .

Notice the little ball near the guy's navel. That is what is called his center of gravity (CG), central point, center of balance, or any other of a host of names. Whatever you call it (I like CG), it is the most important aspect of staying upright. Our entire ability to stay up is tied to that particular point. If it is messed with, our balance is messed with. If our balance is messed with, gravity takes over and we suck earth. It's that simple.

Look at Figure 22. While there are certain exceptions, generally if our CG or upper torso goes outside the cone, we fall over. That is the point of no return I mentioned.

Awwwwww! He Fell Down!

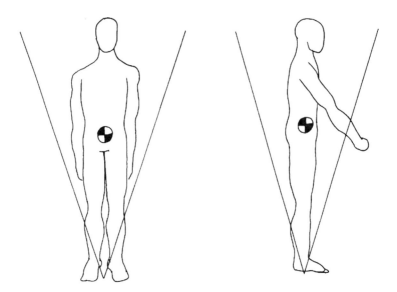

Figure 21. Center of balance.

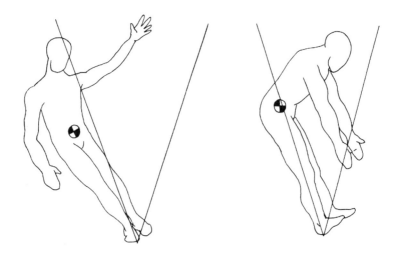

Figure 22. The point of no return.

A Professional's Guide to Ending Violence Quickly

Try this. Stand up and, with your feet close together, try to put your CG into those areas and not fall down. Play around with it for a few minutes. Try it with your shoulders side to side and to the back.

Once you reach this point, there are only two basic ways to keep from going over (Figure 23). One is to counterbalance. Using either a leg, torso, or your ass (which is what happens when you lean forward and touch your toes), you shift your balance to create a compensating opposing weight. The other option is to create a stance that is strong enough to withstand the pull of gravity. Usually this takes half your weight (your legs) and removes it from the equation. The first option is a real delicate balance that can be upset easily, while the second is vulnerable to an incoming force from another direction (Figure 24).

So the answer to any resistance you might encounter while inflicting this law of physics on someone is simply to reapply the same thing in a slightly different direction. Putting it simply, if you encounter resistance coming in one way, just change directions.

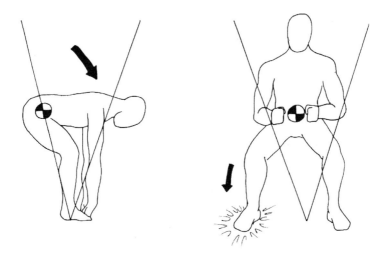

Figure 23. Countermeasures . . .

Awwwwww! He Fell Down!

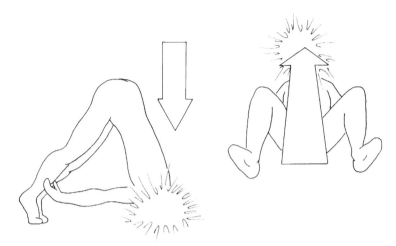

Figure 24. . . . and consequences.

Perhaps the best way to understand it is to think of the guy as inside a funnel that starts from the floor, as shown in the illustrations. What you want to do to get him to lose his balance is to somehow get him outside that funnel. Once he moves outside the funnel's area, gravity pounces on him. The good news is that the more he moves around inside that funnel, the more likely he is to get close to its walls and the less work you have to do to get him over the edge.

Basically, it is easier to throw/drop/pull/shove someone who is moving than it is to do the same to someone who is standing still. If they are moving, they are closer to the edge of the funnel and they're already moving their body weight (Figure 25).

By the way, by the word "easier" I mean you have to apply less force. Yet if the guy is moving, the odds are he's trying to break your face, which some people feel complicates the whole affair, and therefore it no longer qualifies as an "easy situation." Well, nobody said it would be all blondes and blow jobs!

A Professional's Guide to Ending Violence Quickly

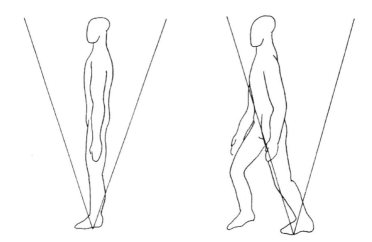

Figure 25.

Now, depending on if the guy is moving full force or if he hasn't really picked up steam generally determines which area you should focus on to take away his balance. From a standing position, or if he just made up his mind that he's "gonna fuck you up" (oooh I'm quiverin' in my boots), your best target is the guy's CG. One good shot here and you're gonna mess up his day big time.

You know, it's funny how years of experience can change a person's perspective. When I was younger I used to be terrified of guys getting right up in my face. I mean, these so-called tough guys would belly right up to me, throw their arms back, and start woofing. It scared me enough that my hand went into my pocket and came out again. I was scared enough of these bully boys that I was about to use a weapon on them.[1] (What struck me as odd was most of the idiots didn't notice that.)

Now when someone tries this on me, the biggest fight I have is to keep from laughing. If you want to guarantee that a guy will move on you, giggle at him while he's doing this tough-guy routine. He will attack, I guarantee it.

Awwwwww! He Fell Down!

The reason that I find this funnier than a Monty Python marathon on a comedy channel is because the guy has just shown me that he is a total fucking amateur! He's standing there with his dick in the microwave trying to impress me with how "bad" he is? I think not! All I have to do is push the "start" button and Nimrod is in for a big surprise. I mean, paint this picture in your head and see if you can keep a straight face.

One of my famous Animal's Laws of Fighting is DON'T CLOSE THE DISTANCE UNTIL YOU ARE ACTUALLY ATTACKING! For professionals you can amend that slightly to, "Don't get close until you've acquired a target and you are getting into position to go for that target." The reason you're standing there is to take him out when he moves. You're not trying to keep him from going off or impress him how tough you are but to take him out. I'm talking targeting the fish eye here. As you're standing there you have a red dot on his center of gravity. When he decides to leap is when you slam him.

I've gone into stance integrity elsewhere. (For those of you who missed it, it's in Appendix F. Learn it, know it, live it.) What I'm going to say here is simply that your best bet for dropping someone fast is to slam into his center of balance from a direction that is perpendicular to his stance integrity, as in Figure 26.

There are four basic reasons why this approach is so effective.

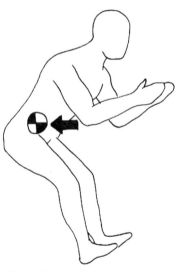

Figure 26.

1) It blows his center of balance down the path of least resistance. We bend forward and backward from the waist easier than side to side.
2) It affects two structural weaknesses of the human body instead of just one: stance integrity and center of gravity. The combination of the two being exploited at once is almost inescapable.
3) Unless the guy is trained to instinctively react to the maneuver, the odds are against him finding the proper counter in time. Besides, if he is trained, the odds are he wouldn't have let you put him into that position in the first place.
4) Most people misinterpret a shot for their center of gravity as an attempted ball shot. By dropping "in" to protect their nuts, not only do they start their body weight moving for you, thereby making your job easier, but they've totally misinterpreted what you were up to. By the time he realizes you weren't going for his gonads, his ass is flying over backward and there ain't a damn thing he can do about it. (Well, you know ol' Sun Tzu did say that all war is based in deception.)

Now let's take a look at something we already discussed—Ye Olde Drop Stepeth. Knoweth that whilst thou may render unto thyne opponent a mighty smite using naught but a body pivot alone, and such wouldst be effective. Wert thou to deliver unto him a mightier smite carried by Ye Olde Drop Stepeth, thoust would surely blow his ass into next weeketh. (Sorry, just got done watching Zepperhelli's *Romeo and Juliet*.)

That's right. If you add a drop step into this move, unless you're real drunk and fighting a granite statue, the guy is going to fold up. If you want to make this even more effective, grab the back of his head while you're moving toward his CG (Figure 27). Not only will most people go "homina homina homina" over which attack to counter (which will allow both to land while dimwit is

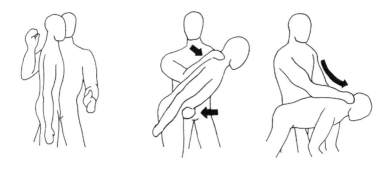

Figure 27.

making up his mind), you can drag his head down faster to guarantee he talks with the ants. I'll explain the downward corkscrew later.

You may have noticed that at this point in the game I haven't mentioned adding in any Attitude Interrupters. Well first off let me point out that the order in which you do this stuff isn't carved in stone. You can do an AI as the guy is going down. (In fact that's exactly what we're going to talk about next.) Secondly, if you did a drop step to blow him over, you've already pressurized his bladder and in a mere moment he's going to encounter terra firma. That's two AIs right there. On many occasions that's going to be enough, and if you're doing this professionally, that's pretty close to the limit of what you're legally supposed to do anyway. But as we all know, shmuck attorneys have left us in a situation where we have a choice: be legal and bleed or be safe and "cross the line into excessive force." (I wonder how long that attitude would last if it was the lawyer facing an enraged drunk and not you.)

Let us for the moment assume that this is just one tough cookie or someone who's seriously lost it. Any witnesses or video cameras? No? Well now let's jes call me a nasty little fucker and pass me them AIs.

There are three reasons why you can lay additional AIs on someone at this point:

1) You're going to butter him up for the biggie that's coming his way. You get him thinking about pain on the way down and he's really going to notice doing a header into the ground. This is real important for getting the attention of drunks and flipouts. Remember what the AI is for—it gets him to change his train of thought.

2) You're really pissed at him for messing up your evening and your chances for getting laid tonight and you want to share your feelings with him. (Of course I've never ever done this. *Snort!*) Maybe not legal, right, or civilized, but it is a common human reaction.

3) You don't think the existing AIs are going to be enough. Someone who's either hard as nails or seriously flipped out—whether from drugs, booze, anger, or mental imbalance—is going to take much more punishment to keep down than someone who's just got a one night's drunk on. If the guy is an experienced fighter, he will know how to handle pain and keep going. Therefore you have to up the volume. The same situation exists for extreme flipouts, but for different reasons. Unlike the tough guy who can ignore the pain, these assholes don't even notice it!

Extreme flipouts don't just happen. There's some serious psychological problems going on with the person, and when they explode it becomes all-consuming. By the time they "flash," nothing else matters except what is spurring them on. A normal person getting drunk and angry is like a campfire, while these people are like bombs. That's why you need to lay in the extra AIs to give them enough stimuli to come back to reality.

At this stage I say that there are two basic ways to apply extra AIs. One is by speeding him on his way and the other is to put crash barriers in his way. A pivot-powered elbow

Awwwwww! He Fell Down!

between the shoulder blades or in the kidney of someone going down gives him something to remember you by during his trip. It also can give him that extra little burst of speed that will make his landing oh so memorable.

Crash barriers are a greatly misunderstood concept. I have met many a young would-be martial artist who had the idea that if the guy is heading toward the earth, they want to punch him so hard that he bounces back up. Why? I don't think that his landing face first is going to hurt the earth.

Generally speaking, I've noticed that these kids seem to have the idea that they want to personally deliver the news to laughing boy that he made a big mistake by messing with them. Don't worry, man, he's going to realize this on his own. You trying to be the first one to tell him can actually end up messing up the full effect. If you hit the guy hard enough to affect him going down, the only thing you've done is slowed him down! He's still going down, regardless of how many martial arts flicks say otherwise. The thing is, now he's not going to hit as hard. So forget hitting the guy so hard that he bounces back up. (Or that you drag him back up and then throw him another way. Don't laugh, I've seen aikidoists do this.) Let him fall.

What you can do is put up a couple of barriers for his face to crash through on the way down. Not only will this add considerable emphasis to the fact that he chose the wrong target for his hostilities, but it also serves as a distraction to keep him from getting ready for his forthcoming landing. You slip in a rattler or two on his way down, whether fist or knee, and you can increase the odds that he's not going to be ready when he hits. You don't have to put that much oomph into them. It's sort of like holding a 2x4 out in front of a speeding motorcycle. It won't exactly stop him, but while he's busy thinking about it, the whole situation is gonna get reeeaaal interesting.

Now I gotta tell you right now—be careful when you use these extras, especially anything that makes him go faster.

Make sure that the situation is serious enough to warrant these sorts of extra moves. The reason is that you can *seriously* hurt someone. If the dude does a header into a fireplug or onto asphalt, he can easily die. That can easily turn into a murder rap. Even if you're a professional, that means your department or company as well as you will end up in court. (Later I will explain some safety nets professionals in high-risk situations can add into all of this to prevent that from happening.)

I also gotta tell you that in some extreme cases, no matter what you do in the AI department, you won't get through. If the guy has gone totally manic on you, there is no way to stop him without doing major structural damage that could permanently cripple or out-and-out kill him unless you've got 14 guys who are willing to get thrown around until you can just dog pile the fucker. Being humane in this case means instead of emptying your magazine into him, you break the fucker's leg and when he tries to get up, you break the other one (and you can bet his lawyers are going to have a field day with that one). If you don't mind getting the shit torn out of you, you could try to choke the guy out, but that's not something I recommend when you're alone.

The bad news is that if you end up facing a manic (or PCP freakout as the media likes to call them, despite the fact that people can and often do reach this state without the help of PCP), no matter what you do to restrain him you run the risk of encountering SDS—Sudden Death Syndrome.

First off, one thing people in manic episodes hate is being restrained. They flip out even worse when you try to restrain them. Secondly, a manic episode pumps enough adrenaline into a person's system to sterilize a bull. The flood gates are wide open, and there is no controlling the epinephrine being dumped into the body. That's what gives the guy superhuman strength. He's basically running on million octane gas. Unfortunately, our little hearts and minds can't handle this sort of strain. Whether it's a heart attack or his nervous system goes "FFFHHHHPT!" like old wiring, the guy just up and dies! It's not because you did any structural damage but because he burned himself out. Guess when this is most likely to happen? When he's restrained. Fuck.

The only good news about all of this is that when someone goes this far south, unless you're a professional you can do the smart thing and just get the hell out of there. There's nothing to be gained by hanging around and trying to handle this sort of situation. The average person is not likely to run into these people, anyway, which makes life oh so much easier.

Now, back to my original point (and yes, I do have one). Most ways to get control of someone's center of gravity are based in the push/impact move. Whether from up front or behind, you're slamming into the guy's CG and knocking it out of kilter. Whether you use your hand or your hip to impact, it all plays the same. Incidentally, the reason this works is because you are not only taking his balance away, you're removing his support. In moving his center of balance out toward the funnel's edge, you're removing what his torso, arm, and head weight were resting on. You've pulled the rug out, and they're going to come crashing down. On top of all this, you've hit him catiwhompus to his stance integrity. For being so simple it is a nasty fucking move.

From behind the technique changes slightly. Why do I mention behind, you may ask? Simple. If you're a professional and you have a partner, he can be talking and distracting the dude while you quietly slip up from behind or the side. If the guy looks at you, just gesture and glance toward your partner as if to say, "Hey you're talking to him, not me." The truth is, while your partner is talking you're the biggest threat. But he doesn't need to know that; just you and your partner do.

There are a couple of ways to do this. Most of them have to do with size—yours and his—but the process is the same in both: you blow the guy's CG and you drag him back over. Unlike from the front, you *need* to use your other hand to take him down from behind. This is because humans don't normally bend this way, and you're moving against a stronger muscle group. If you don't do this fast enough, the guy will be able to resist effectively. That hand is there to make sure he doesn't get the chance to resist.

For a bigger guy on a smaller or same-size opponent, you step in (using a drop step, naturally) and, with your weaker hand, swat/shove his CG forward. Meanwhile your stronger hand has glommed onto his shoulder or you've put your forearm across the top of his sternum (which is better) and you're pulling him backward and down from his shoulder (Figure 28). What this does is catch him

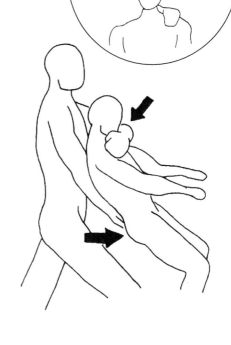

Figure 28.

between two opposing forces on different levels and turn an area around his short ribs into a pivot with his body weight trying to go horizontal.

If the guy gets antsy about you being behind him, you can do the same thing from the side, although it is a little harder and the guy can slip out of your hands like a Vaseline-coated catfish. Not that he'll go far, but it won't be a controlled fall. From the side, you again do a drop step to his back while catching him on the shoulder. Add in a pivot and slam your hand into his center of gravity (Figure 29).

To help keep the guy from catfishing away from you, clothesline him with your forearm across his collarbone, then slide it across to where you can turn it into a neck hold if necessary. Incidentally, for most of these moves it's best to position yourself off the guy's right shoulder. For one thing, most people aren't trained fighters, so it's unlikely that they'll be able to muster an attack with any juice before you take them. Secondly, you're jamming their strong side. Generally, it's easier to take someone forward from a side position (or to do my personal favorite and take his support away), but this side back drop is still a good thing to have up your sleeve in case things get weird.

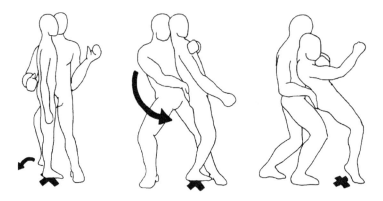

Figure 29.

A minor complication exists when it's a smaller guy who needs to take out a bigger guy this way. It can be done, but you need to know a few points.[2] The fundamental difference is you have to do something that I normally hate to advise: you gotta leave the ground. Literally, you may have to jump on the fucker's back. However, there are ways to do it and ways to do it. One will end up with you getting tossed around like a rag doll, while the other will end up with him on the ground.

The reason you have to leapfrog is because a bigger guy has more body mass, and you're going to need as much of yours as possible to get him moving. The other difference is you may need to use both hands on his shoulders. If the guy is only slightly bigger, you can get away with doing the same-size sort of moves I've already discussed. If the guy is just taller than you without much mass, you can get away with maybe one hand on his shoulder while the other paddles his CG. If the guy is seriously taller than you, you may want to consider using one hand to slam his CG while grabbing his hair and dragging it back. It's a harder target to get a hold of before he reacts (even with long hair), but if you're quick, oftentimes you can do this rather than the forthcoming alternative.

If the dude is way bigger than you, it can get ugly. You have to literally knee him in the back while pulling him down. This puts you into position to gain control of his fall. The problem is that the SOB's center of gravity can be seriously higher than your hips! In this case you have to leap up with your knee extended and slam it into his CG. As you're bouncing off, grab his shoulders with both hands and drag him over backward. It's kind of like intentionally bouncing off a wall. You don't want to drive his entire body forward, just his CG. Meanwhile, your entire body weight is sliding down his back, pulling his shoulders over and down (Figure 30).

The hard part is that you have to land in such a way that you can catch the gorilla's falling body weight, which means

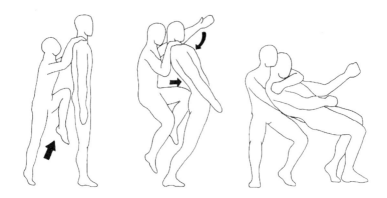

Figure 30.

in a wide-legged stance with your thigh under there. Your arm will be doing a lot of the work, but that thigh is important backup to catch the galoot. And let's not forget snaking that arm around the top of his sternum now, shall we?[3]

By the way, this move takes a shitload of practice, namely because it has to be done *fast*. If you don't take the guy's CG upon impact, he's going to throw your ass around like a rag doll! This move is only recommended in situations where you have to restrain the dude rather than let him go into a freefall (for example, if you are an ER orderly with a Saturday night freakout and administration would get pissed if you just hit him over the head with a bottle of saline).

This brings up a very important point. I will deal with this more extensively in Chapter 11, but right now I want to point out that there is a difference between what a professional has to do and what you can do as a private citizen. In many ways a professional is more restricted than a private citizen. If this guy attacks you, as a private citizen you are expected to be less competent regarding self-defense than if you are a professional. If you are a professional, you are expected to be able to restrain the guy before you resort to stronger means. While you can get in trouble in both cases for being better at violence than the asshole who attacked you, a professional has to have higher standards about use of force than the average civilian because he is constantly facing it! He cannot just let the guy fly off into space to land on whatever.

A pro must first try to restrain, then do a controlled fall (with the option of restraining at any time), and only last can he let the guy go into a freefall. Putting that in English, that means he's got to 1) wrestle the dude, 2) judo/jujutsu him, and finally, if nothing else works, 3) just drop the SOB on his head. For those of you who are not professionals, still keep this standard in mind, as it can lessen your chances of ending up in court over some drunk asshole.

While blowing the guy's CG out into left field will generally start him moving downward, there are a few things that you can do to aid and abet this process. Namely, grab something important that's falling and speed up its descent. The back of the guy's head is one of my personal favorites (although shoulders and backs also work).

Ever watch a drunk walk? Take what I'm about to tell you and go see for yourself. The inner ear resides where? In the head. It is from our inner ear where we find our balance. A drunk is like someone walking with a bowl of water on his head. His entire body will shift around trying to keep his head (and inner ear) level. That's because if it moves too much he's going to lose his balance and fall over! Seriously, watch someone walk who is plowed. His entire body is stumbling around beneath his head trying to keep his head in one place!

Go take a look at Figure 21 again and take a guess what would happen if the guy's head got outside of that funnel. Now guess what happens if you grab his head and drag it out into the point of no return for him. Exactly! Now the best way to do this is, after you've stepped up and delivered an AI or two to the guy and blown his CG to hell, go back to a concept I mentioned back in Chapter 3. That is Option D—force bouncing back from an object it encounters.

Awwwwww! He Fell Down!

Let's say that you've delivered a serious drop step AI and blown the dude's center of gravity out the window. Do you want to stand there and let him fall on you? Of course not! So what you do is take the rebound energy of your last shot to the guy and turn it into another drop step . . . only this time backward! Not only does this get you out of the way of laughing boy's trip to the ground (after all, who are

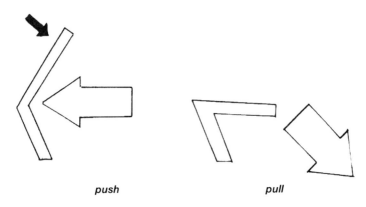

push *pull*

Figure 31.

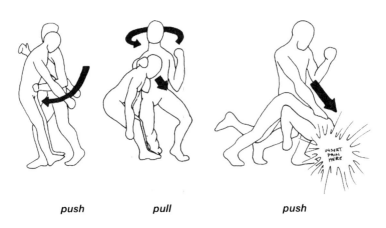

push *pull* *push*

Figure 32.

A Professional's Guide to Ending Violence Quickly

we to interfere with gravity?), but the action of grabbing his head while stepping back also allows you to add a little zest to his trip.

In this particular move you want your body weight to weigh heavily on him heading down rather than moving forward. Unlike your first move, instead of your body weight pushing against him, you're now pulling, as in Figure 31.

Since you've already moved his ass toward the edge of the funnel, any extra weight on him is going to rocket him past the edge and into Mamasan Terra Firma. As you step away, grab whatever is available and shove it down. Since you are flexing your knees while you're stepping, your entire body weight is behind that hand on the back of the guy's head. Once the guy is past you, throw in a pivot and straighten your arm. By the way, at this point you've suddenly shifted back to pushing again (Figure 32).

Oh by the way, always be sure to grab an area that doesn't stretch. That way your body weight can't be absorbed. A head only goes so far. Shoulders too. But grabbing a guy's wrist when his arm is bent allows him to straighten his arm and removes the effectiveness of your weight being used to speed him on the way down. I'll talk about this more in the slaving chapter.

So basically, one of the best ways to take someone to the ground is to push against his center of gravity and grab his head/shoulders. It's quick, it's fast, and it's effective. However sometimes there just isn't enough room or time to do that, so we are just going to have to mess around with a few more options.

ENDNOTES

1. A combination of the rules of my upbringing: "Don't carry unless you're willing to pull it, don't pull it unless you're willing to use it, don't use it unless you're willing to kill with it." A bad experience with flashing a faulty switchblade when I was 10 and some hardcore training with an experienced street fighter taught me not to

flash weapons. Always watch the fucker who holds his hand down by his side.

2. I used to love coming out of a group of huge bouncers who were facing off a drunk and them stepping back and saying to the dude, "He's the head man." The drunk would look at little me, then big them, and back to little me and know something wasn't quite right there.

3. It's always important to remember to take a guy down by an arm across the collarbone/sternum rather than across his neck/throat. While you can always shift over to a chokehold after you take him down, it is way too easy to seriously hurt the dude doing a takedown via his throat . . . and that means lawyers.

CHAPTER 7

There's More'n One Way to Skin a Cat

"If it's stupid, but it works, it isn't stupid."
—Murphy's Laws of Combat #2

While taking control of the guy's center of gravity is one of the better ways to take him down, there are less sophisticated ways that you may have to resort to—namely, just blowing the sucker over. Much of this can be related to slaving him to the effects of gravity on your body, or it can be as simple as just slamming into him against his line of stance integrity.

Remember Ook, the Neanderthal martial arts master from *Floor Fighting*? Well, not only was Ook the inventor of the AK-1 (a large rock) and the gorilla grip, but he also gave us one of the most basic ways to take someone's balance away from them. That is, to simply tackle the fucker.

While some could conceivably argue that this is more a matter of slaving someone to the effects of gravity on you, I can tell you from personal experience that if you don't hit the dude hard enough to blow him off balance, he ain't going nowhere. I've had a wide array of experiences, and believe me, few of them were less fun than trying to tackle someone with no effect in the middle of a fight.

Two major things have an effect here. One is his weight vs. your weight, and the second, most importantly, is how fast you are moving when you hit him. Basically, the less you weigh compared to him, the faster you have to be moving to compensate for his greater mass.[1] This is especially true if you hit him up near his chest instead of doing the smart thing and tackling him at his center of gravity. Remember your high school football coach: "Hit him low!"

Personally, unless the guy is alone and you aren't, I seriously don't recommend going down to the ground with the dude, which is why I'm sort of hesitant about a tackle, but sometimes you just have no choice. I wrote an entire book about this subject (*Floor Fighting*, if you haven't caught on yet), and if you're interested in continuing breathing, I recommend you read it, especially if you've been trained in nice traditional techniques. It's biting-ears-off time in that book, and that's what you're going to be meeting in the streets.

One trick I learned recently (by having the guy try and pull it on me, thank you very much) is, as you're going down with the dude, grab a handful of his hair on the back of his head and pull back so his head hits the ground. Now mind you this is a dirty, low-down, despicable street fighter's trick that can possibly result in the guy dying. (Then again, it also happened to be a dirty, low-down, despicable street fighter who was attempting to pull it on me, so he wasn't really concerned with my safety at the time.) If it hadn't had been for the fact that I always instinctively curl up as I fall, that trick would have worked. As it was, all it did was leave my scalp tender for a couple of days.

Twisting so your shoulder lands in the guy's rib cage is loads of laughs. And of course, no party would be complete without that added elbow in his solar plexus. If you're feeling particularly vicious and aren't really concerned if the guy

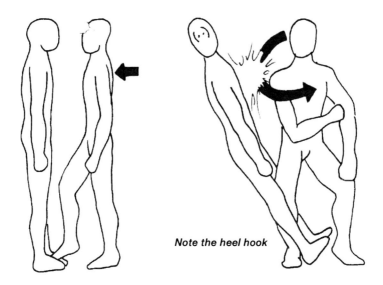

Note the heel hook

Figure 33. Shoulder slam.

stays in this plane of existence, you can always lay your forearm across his throat. When that old street fighter and I went over, by God we used all of these. It was an ugly moment.

Let us for a moment assume you'd like to think that you're a little past Ook's level. You're more interested in making sure the other guy goes down alone. Okay, let's go then to phase two.

Ever notice how fights tend to get up close real quick? I mean, there you are slugging it out, and the next moment you're right up close and nearly kissing. Uncool, this. You ain't got no room to effectively hit the dude, but you're still locked up.

However, did you know that from this nearly impossible position, with the simple application of something I mentioned earlier (and hopefully you've been practicing), you can blow the guy off his feet without actually hitting him? If you were to happen to throw in an elbow you could blend this with an AI.

There's More'n One Way to Skin a Cat

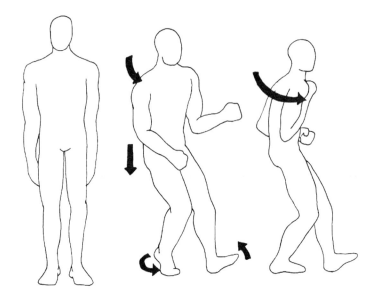

Figure 34. The corkscrew.

The move I'm talking about is the pivot/drop step. Yep, yep, yep, yep. Remember what you saw earlier—energy coming in one direction, then changing to come in perpendicular against the guy's stance integrity. It's the same thing, except instead of a shove you shoulder-check the guy (Figure 33). That means your shoulder slams into the center of his chest. From point-blank range you can knock someone on his ass.

Needless to say, having the timing down between your pivot and drop step so everything gets there at once really does help. You also can throw in an elbow at this time to make it less fun. (Besides, at that close none of the witnesses are really going to see exactly what happened.)

Sometimes you can't get in a full drop step, so what you have to do is corkscrew. Basically, a corkscrew is when you just collapse your knees and start falling straight down. In the middle of this you slap in a pivot, lift your heels, tuck

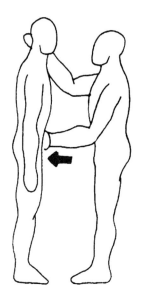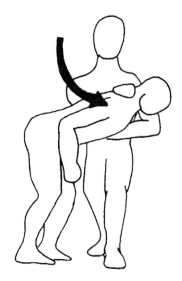

Figure 35. Corkscrew pull.

your shoulder forward, and tighten your knees. When your shoulder hits, it's going to come in with all the force of your falling body.

This particular motion has lots of clout in a very small area and has multiple uses both when pushing and pulling. If you glom onto the back of someone's head and twist downward like this, add a downward jerk onto it with your arm (Figure 35). I've dragged over much bigger opponents who, until then, had been absolutely sure they were about to overwhelm me with their superior size and strength. Of course if you're that close you can just head-butt the shmuck.

Now stepping back a little, if you land an open-hand drop step/pivot into your opponent's centerline, you have just found one of the few effective strikes to the chest (Figure 36). It's better to do this open-handed, as you're less likely to break your wrist against the guy's entire body weight.

There's More'n One Way to Skin a Cat

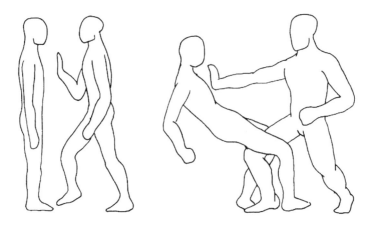

Again with this heel hook thing

Figure 36. Drop step/open-hand strike.

While any of these can be delivered from up front, they are generally more effective when you've slipped off the line of attack. (Like onto his 45; remember that?) This is because they are circular motions, and they come in from an unexpected direction.

However, sometimes the guy will be standing in front of you. Remember the idiot with the puffed-up chest standing right in front of you? I have sent many of them ass over tea kettle with a simple drop-step, double-palm strike (Figure 37).

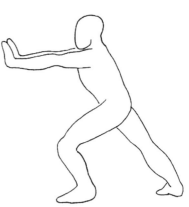

Figure 37. Drop step/double-palm strike.

Naturally, if there is some kind of table, chair, or low wall behind him, it's going to get kind of entertaining. For those situations where that is not enough and he hasn't gone down, a quick front snap kick to his nuts as he's backpedaling trying to regain his balance will really mess up his concentration, hence his balance. If it did work and he looks like he's dumb enough to try and get up, just kick him in the face to convince him how stupid that idea is. Of course if he tries to get up by rolling over, a quick drop punch to his kidneys is just as effective. If this goes against your sense of fair play, you can warn him not to try to get up before you sucker punch him.

Needless to say, all of these can be utilized from behind. Since we normally walk forward, however, as with any action that throws the guy that way, it's more likely that he will regain his balance by running real fast so his feet catch up to his head. So don't forget to either shove him toward something (preferably something low) or at least hook his foot as you shove.

Now for you sneaky SOBs, one of my personal favs is the side drop step/ elbow strike. Although this can be used to suddenly screw up someone's day when you're standing there look-ing innocent, I really like it when some slick little fuck does what I like to do and ghosts to the side while his partner distracts you from the front. Not only does it give the ghost a hard time, but it sets you up for a per-fect hook into the talker.

What it is is a drop step to the side, very much like the first experimental drop step I had you do. From a standing position, simply lift one leg and fall to the

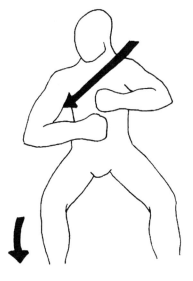

Figure 38. Side drop/elbow.

side, add in some kick from your other foot, and drive your elbow out to the side (Figure 38). All you need to do to throw a hook from here is pivot.

Not only does this slam the ghost a real good one, but if you drop low enough you're slamming into his CG. Keep this one in mind for situations where there's a shark grinning at you and being totally civil as he's trying to get into attack position. It's also great fun to do on drunk assholes at cocktail parties. Do it fast enough and while no one else is looking and you can claim you stumbled. Needless to say, you should watch for this one being pulled on you while you're standing to the side waiting to drop the putz.

One thing I'd like to mention here, but it applies to any and all forward takedowns, is what you can do to make them more effective. Like I said earlier, in forward takedowns the guy is likely going to be able to run fast enough to have his feet sort of catch up to him. If this doesn't save him entirely, it can at least serve as a means to slow his descent. In other words, his descent can end up looking like Figure 39.

Basically what happens is that by falling in segments, A) he's not going to hit as hard as if he were to go down directly, and B) he doesn't get hurt as bad. By running, he bleeds off the energy of his descent into another motion. That means his downward descent is arrested and instead of hitting the ground from 6+ feet, the next stage of his fall will be

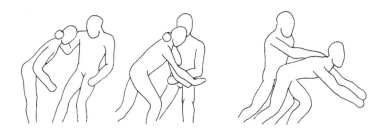

Figure 39.

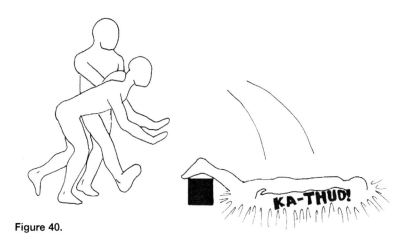

Figure 40.

only from 3 or so feet (unless he happens to run into a table or wall during his horizontal forward phase). This is why you need to stick a foot out there if you want his fall to be an AI (Figure 40). Of course if you're a professional who's only trying to contain the guy without damaging him too much, you should reserve this tripping trick only for the biggest assholes . . . er . . . I mean the most violent individuals.

In a related vein, what is the instinctive reaction when you fall down? Yeah, you put your hands up to catch yourself. Why? Because it works. Your hands and arms serve as a great big shock absorber to slow you down and keep you from slamming into Mother Earth (whereas a trained gymnast, contact sport athlete, fighter, or stuntman will add in a body twist too).

Now if this works so well at keeping you from hitting the ground too hard, what naturally don't you want the guy you're throwing around like a sack of potatoes to do? That's right, you don't want him to get his arms up there to catch him. If he does, he's going to miss the full effect of the neat trick you just did.

So here's the trick. You need to do something that momentarily renders the guy's arms ineffective for catching him. I've broken a guy's arm before I knocked him over, but that may be a little too intense for some of you. Naturally, if you take him over backwards he's not going to be able to do much to catch himself. This combined with the feet not working so well in that direction is why I prefer taking people over backwards myself, in spite of the higher risk of him breaking his head open. But that's my own way of doing things, and I instinctively go to protect his head when I do this. You have to find what works for you.

One of the really effective points of all those jujutsu kind of wrist and arm locks is that they automatically tie up one of the guy's hands. With one hand tied up, at best he's only going to be able to do half the job of catching himself.[2] More often than not, the guy is going to be so confused about what is going on that he won't be able to get that free hand up in time to do anything effective, even though it is free. See Figure 20 for a visual refresher.

In a similar situation, what you can do with the very hand that you checked his attack with is hold it down long enough (or shove it aside hard enough) that the same effect is achieved. Your checking hand prevents him from getting his hand up fast enough to catch himself. In other words, by leaving that hand there for a second or two longer than normal, you can make sure the guy hits about five times harder. Good return on your investment, I'd say.

ENDNOTES

1. In my book *Pool Cues, Beer Bottles, and Baseball Bats*, I give an in-depth explanation of the physics of smaller/lighter vs. bigger/ heavier situations. If your mind works that way, with this formula you can pick up any weapon and know how you'll have to move to make it more effective.

2. By the way, while many people are under the false impression that I'm down on these "wrestling" arts for real fighting, let me assure you that I'm not. They are stone-cold perfect for finishing work. Often we don't pay enough attention to the ending of a situation,

but it is just as, if not more important than the beginning. While the guy walking point may be getting more glamour, the guy who's bringing up the rear (the sweeper) is going to be the dude who saves your ass when it gets thick. My only problem with these arts is based on timing. Don't rush to get into position to use these kind of moves, because there's a whole lot of shit you can do before you need to get in their effective range.

There's More'n One Way to Skin a Cat

CHAPTER 8

Taking Away His Support

"To be certain to take what you attack is to attack a place the enemy does not protect. To be certain to hold what you defend is to defend a place where the enemy does not attack."

—Sun Tzu
The Art of War

There are three fundamental ways to take away someone's support:

1) Collapse it.
2) Blow it out from underneath him.
3) Snag it up. What all this means is you take his two points of support and suddenly reduce it to one, thereby leaving his wobbly ass hanging out there and subject to the whims of gravity. Not too complicated, is it?
Look at how someone normally stands, then notice

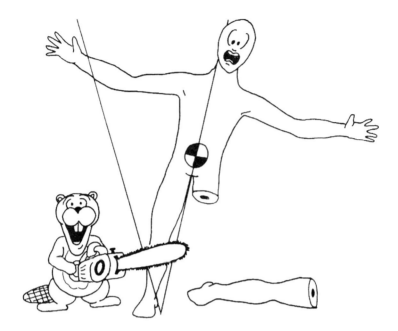

Figure 41.

what happens when you take one of the supports away (without him shifting to compensate). You will observe that the guy's center of gravity is already at the point of no return. Which way does gravity work? Which way is he going? Which way are you going to help him go with a well-placed yank on the shoulder or shove? (Hint: they all start with the letter D.)

Each of these three ways can seem to be sort of repeating each other, but they are distinct actions. Just in passing, however, I should point out that they do work best in combination, which might be what leads to the confusion. Let me explain.

Collapsing someone's support basically means that you do something that causes the guy's leg to buckle. Suddenly something happens that makes his leg collapse under him, and before he can reestablish his support, gravity has done

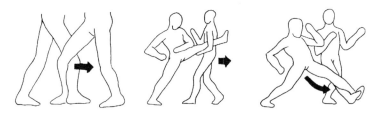
Figure 42. Blowing out his support.

its dirty deed. Of all the moves, this happens to be the easiest and fastest. This usually means that you do something like dropping your knee into his and causing his leg to fold. Or if you want to be more spectacular, you break the guy's kneecap and watch him fall over.

Blowing someone's support out from underneath him means that you do some action that either drags or shoves his leg/foot out from beneath him (Figure 42). Things like the illustrious Tiger Tail Sweep are what most people think of when I mention this move. I prefer simple things like hooking the guy's foot with yours as you're stepping back so he falls into the splits (and rips all sorts of interesting things) or, one of my all-time favorites, catching kicks and just stepping back while lifting up. Simpler, and they don't leave you as exposed if things go wrong as the tiger sweep.

There are two ways to do this particular kind of move: the hard way or the easy way. The hard way is to go after the load-bearing foot and knock it out from underneath him. Unless the dude is on a slippery surface, though, this can be sort of difficult. If you're a lazy fuck like myself, you can either go after one foot when his weight is equally divided (hence having to only move half the load) or, my personal favorite, just snake on in when he steps and blow aside what will in about a second become a load-bearing leg. The guy goes to put his weight on his support and it ain't there no mo! Too late to stop it now, hombre!

Naturally, you can do the same thing going in the other direction too—that is, you don't have to go outward, you

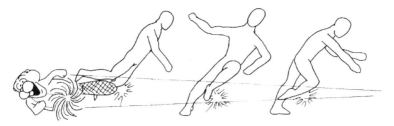

Figure 43. Blowing support inward.

can go inward. Two things complicate this one, though: 1) you have to be fast enough to make sure the guy can't regain his balance by putting his foot down closer, and 2) the fucker might fall on you. It sort of helps to slip to the side and out of the guy's path of descent (remembering to block any attempts to latch onto support). Snagging someone's support is basically tripping the dude. You lock his feet up so he can't move either when he's in the process of moving (so his own momentum carries him onto his face) or before you slam into him.

Now I would like to point something out here. Our little friend, Mr. Busy Beaver, was specifically chosen to point something out to you. Ol' BB there managed to take out an opponent many times his size. You will notice that he never struck against his opponent's superior body weight; rather, he pitted his weight against the weight of his opponent's support leg. I don't care who you are, even if you're a tiny 5-foot nothin' 99-pound wisp of a girl, you're still heavier than the guy's leg! If you throw your weight at that target, his big burly 250 pounds is going to become his problem right quick. That's because all of it is going to be heading to the ground and picking up speed as it goes!

As you can see, none of these are particularly complicated theories. The most difficult thing to do is to start thinking about your feet. Or is that on your feet? Anyway, it's paying attention to your footwork and his. Not something that most people generally pay much attention too.

Want to know a great way to learn how to move your feet quickly into weird positions, "think" with your feet, and practice accuracy with your feet?

Ever seen a group of tie-dyed long-haired hippie types standing around in a circle? How about a group of college students doing the same? If they are jumping around, the odds are that they are playing a game called Hacky Sack. Hacky Sack is a very old European game made popular again by thousands and thousands of stoned Renaissance Festival types over the last 30 years. Since many of them are Dead Heads and college students, you can see where the connection would come in.

Hacky Sack basically consists of kicking around a small leather ball. Like soccer, you can't use your hands. Unlike soccer, the sack can't touch the ground. In fact the object of the game it to keep the ball in the air for as long as possible. It works best with about four or five players, but you can practice by yourself or with another person. You can get the sacks at any toy store (tell anyone who's asking that you're getting it for a relative if you're embarrassed). Be forewarned: it's harder than you think to keep it going for any length of time. But it's fun. That's why it's such a good exercise to teach you about your footwork. By the way, don't think your normal martial arts are going to help on this one. I did and boy was I embarrassed. (Since it is not obviously related to kicking the shit out of someone, you can probably get your old lady to play. Great way to spend time with your sweetie at the park, have fun, and practice all rolled into one.)

So let's go look at collapsing the guy's support for a second. Like the man said in the movie *Roadhouse*, "It don't matter how big a guy is, you take his knee out . . ." We learn early that most big guys have clay feet and particleboard knees.

The easiest way to collapse someone's knee is to simply fold it the way that it normally goes. That means you hit the back of the knee and start it folding. Unless the guy has his leg muscles locked up, it's not going to take much to start

Taking Away His Support

the process (and if he does have it locked up, well then it's much easier just to bust than to try and fold).

There are several ways to collapse someone's knee in this manner. One is to do a drop step into the back of his knee with the front of yours. The other one is to lift your foot up and just step onto the top of his calf and through the back of his knee (Figure 44). The course your body mass is following is diagonally down and forward. This blows his support out from underneath him, carries him with you (slaving him to you) downward, and makes it real hard for him to get his leg out from underneath yours and out in front to catch himself. If you have to be nice, it lets you turn his fall into a slide along your leg, which keeps him from hitting as hard.

Generally speaking, the knee drop works best for opponents who are the same size or larger than you, whereas the step seems to work for bigger guys taking down smaller opponents. In either case, you can let the dude fall or grab him and hold him a hair past the point of no return.

Now a third variation is reaching down and just slapping or karate chopping the back of the guy's knee. While all of these knee folds work better with a downward pulling

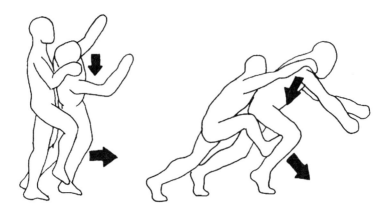

Figure 44. Collapsing the knee.

hand on the guy's shoulder to take him down faster, this one requires it. You might want to do this if you are in a profession where you have to do controlled takedowns. If done right (read: fucking fast and hard), it gives you better control over the guy's body weight, thereby giving you the ability to either keep him suspended or control his fall so he doesn't hurt himself. Unfortunately if done wrong (read: too slow and not hard enough), you're going to catch an elbow in the face at the very least.

Generally speaking, I recommend using your legs to collapse his support until you get good enough at dropping people quickly. Then you might want to consider using the hand chop versions shown in Figure 45. While the hand jobs are less likely to hurt the dude, they're more likely to get you hurt.

Another variation comes about when you're dealing with one of those chumps who has legs like tree trunks. I'm talking about those goons who have knees like a bull. No shit, I've seen guys who were 6'2" who had knees lower than mine. Not a fun person to try and drive his knee into the ground. This can apply with fat guys.

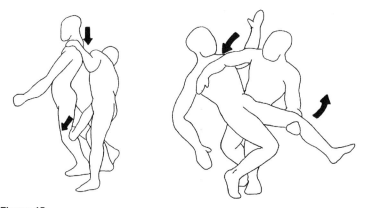

Figure 45.

Taking Away His Support

In cases like this, what you can do is basically sweep up his knee (Figure 46). When you hit the back of his knee with yours, you bring your knee up in an arc as if you're trying to touch it to your chest. What you've done is lifted his leg up instead of dropping it down. While this is technically more a category 2 move of blowing his support aside, it is applicable here. Take his knee up with your leg and either shove or pull with your hands. If you shove you have to follow him for awhile, holding up his knee so he can't regain his balance by putting his foot down until it's too late. If you pull, either be ready to catch him or scurry like a rabbit to keep from getting crushed as he falls on you. This move has to be done in a drop step manner, as you really gotta slam hard into these kinds of guys.

Now while what I've been showing you works the best from behind, it can also be done from the side. Granted it's safer and more effective from behind, but unless the guy's real drunk or dumb he'll notice you cruising behind him. (Oddly enough, though, most violence involves drunk and dumb people, so there you go.)

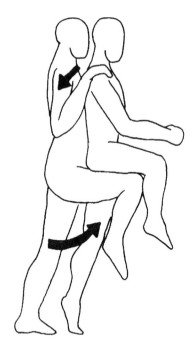

Again, we look at what you can do from the side. One is to stand off to the guy's right (remember, less swinging power there) and if it gets ugly do a cork-screw/pivot on your right leg and drive your knee into his leg. (Keep your right side away from the dude if you carry a gun.) Then,

Figure 46. Knee lift.

with your hands, either drive him down or over backwards (Figure 47). Believe it or not, this is one of the few times that you don't want everything landing at once. The action of your knee is going one direction while the downward shove/pull is going another. It gets real messy if you try to do it all at once. However plowing into the dude's leg and *then* pivoting the other way in either a drag or a forearm across the upper chest works well. If it sounds awkward and complicated, that's because it is.

This is another one of those "can't I just hurt the asshole?" kind of moves that can get you hurt while trying not to harm the aggressor to keep you or your department from getting sued. It's really sort of clumsy, but it allows you to control his fall. In the same vein, the back of the knee slap I mentioned earlier can work more easily and more effectively from this position, although you are still risking that damned elbow. However both of these keep your gun out of reach while you're trying to subdue someone without hurting him—someone who would happily shoot you if he got his hands on your gun.

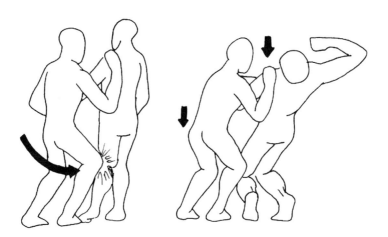

Figure 47.

Taking Away His Support

Now let's say that you're slightly less concerned about hurting the guy >:-D (Internet sign for evil laugh). At this point, the easiest thing for you to do is to just slam your knee into the outside of his, driven by a drop step. For those of you who cannot use excessive force, know that A) few people will actually be able to tell the difference where you hit while watching, and B) you can always claim that you were aiming for the back of his knee and he moved. Hard to prove otherwise.

The thing about the knee is that, next to bending it in the normal fashion, the easiest way to buckle someone's leg is by driving the knee inward toward its partner. The reason is that the entire leg rotates inward easier than it does outward. Once this leg rotation has happened, then the knee just bends in the normal fashion. You're still getting the same bend, just now the leg is in a different position.

The guy will usually try to roll instinctively with a force coming in on the side of his knee. As he's rolling and pivoting to keep from getting a broken leg, he automatically puts himself into a position where his leg will buckle. If that isn't on a silver platter, I don't know what is.

Depending on how far to the back of the guy's knee you were, the more likely he is to fold without breaking. Also, how much your force is heading in alignment to the way his knee normally folds tends to lessen the chances of breakage. If you come in with a hard-core thrust kick to the side of the knee, it's likely to snap like a twig, whereas a knee slamming into the rear area of his knee can and will force him to twist around and fall over.

The closer you are to coming in straight from the side, the more likely you are to snap his knee. While it can be done with a knee drop, a step kick or side thrust kick is the best way to smash a knee. Needless to say, if you don't want to be that savage, take care not to come in from this angle. If you do want to be this savage, take care to come in from this angle.

Now oddly enough, if you come in off an oblique front angle (like a slip/drop step to avoid the guy's attack), you

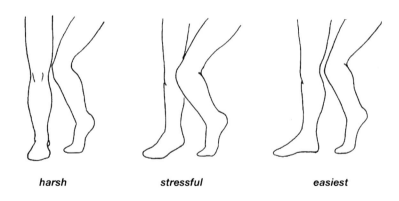

harsh   *stressful*   *easiest*

Figure 48. Bending the knee.

are in a better position to buckle his knee than to break it. The reason is that the knee is harder to break from the front than it is from the side. Why? Because that's how the muscles, joints, and tendons are rigged so we can walk. If the guy's knee is bent at all, you're going to cause it to roll inward before it's in any danger of breaking. So jam that leg up!

When you come in with your drop step, be sure to slam your tensed-up leg into that guy's outer knee. It makes for loads of laughs when the guy realizes he just got his leg kicked aside as well as his chimes rung (Figure 49).

Something else you might want to remember in a situation like this is that most people don't have the experience to make sure everything lands at once. Unlike you, his body weight may not be slamming down at the exact second his punch reaches it destination. In fact, odds are that it's a second or two behind. So a lot of times you can get in there before the guy has put his weight on that leg. And that, my friends, is very close to the next point of blowing someone's support out from underneath him!

I learned the stamp kick from wing chun (wing tsun for you purists). Not only was it a great way to buckle a knee,

Taking Away His Support

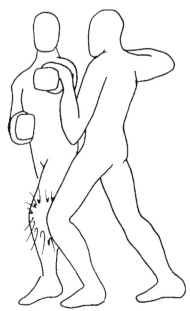

Figure 49.

but it made for great blocks against most kicks. If the guy starts any kind of front or roundhouse kick, you just stomp on it! Pfffttttt! Forget that move, Charlie! It's faster than most kicks since you're actually kicking toward his foot or ankle as it leaves the ground; you're not losing time by trying to gain altitude. He's trying to bring his foot up and you're stomping down on it. This can be done to the front or the sides.

The reason I mention this is twofold. If the guy is an inexperienced kicker or drunk, he can easily make the mistake of committing his weight into the kick, not tighten his foot, or kick with his toe first. If you take his kick on the sole of your foot (Figure 51) you can either cause him to fall over (rare) or break his foot or toe (common). His ability to handle pain will determine whether he just hobbles around or falls over when he tries to put weight on it again. I've broken more than one person's foot using this

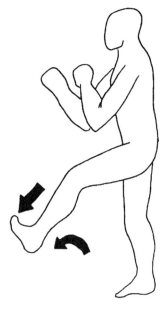

Figure 50. Stamp kick.

A Professional's Guide to Ending Violence Quickly

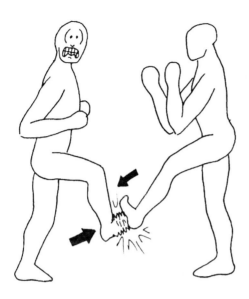

Figure 51.

technique, namely because by stomping on their kick I catch them before they can prepare. They often haven't tensed for impact yet. Even if they curled their toes back, I'm landing right on them.

The second reason I mention this kind of kick is because it is absolutely perfect for kicking someone's leg out from underneath him in the middle of his step, especially the side-to-side version. While the guy is taking a step, you just snake on in and whap it out of the way. Suddenly the support that he was expecting to be there to catch him ain't.

Remarkably, it is more effective to kick the guy's leg in what is called an inverse direction than anything else. Inversion means inwards, sorta. Actually it means 90 degrees off how it normally bends, but in an inwardly direction. Depending on where the guy's foot is at the time sort of changes which way "inward" is, which is why I can't use that term. Inverse, however, doesn't change.

If you try to kick it out in the opposite direction (eversion), he can usually widen his stance to compensate. Since you're kicking instead of pulling, you're more likely to run out of leg before he does. All of which means he's still standing, he's now closer to you, and he's probably more pissed that you just tried to sucker him.

Taking Away His Support

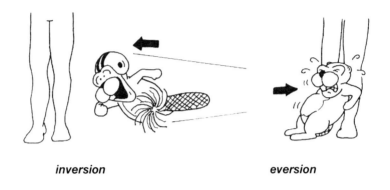

inversion   *eversion*

Figure 52. Inversion vs. eversion.

You can run into problems trying to kick the guy's foot backward if his toe/ball of his foot drags out. You try to kick it backward and instead you just force him to put his foot down near where it was when he started. Nah, not good enough. In order to compensate for this likelihood, you have to lift his foot, which is better to do with a hook/pull than a push (which I'll explain later).

One of the real problems with trying to move the guy's foot from the eversion direction with a kick is that you are more likely to run out of your leg before he reaches the point where his leg is knocked out from underneath him. Also, if you're kicking that way, you're leg is likely to be underneath him when he falls. Sounds stupid, but I was once involved in a situation where it happened.

However, if you kick or sweep the guy's foot in an inverse direction, as in Figure 53, you buckle his leg in a way that is a bitch to recover from. There are several reasons for this. Number one, he's going to run out of balance long before you run out of leg to keep pushing. Number two, you're there between him and solid footing. Number three, you can lift to keep his foot from ever hitting the ground.

Here's the real rub of all of this. Unless the guy knows to lift his foot up high and shake you loose or immediately

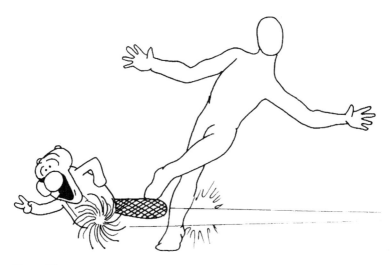

Figure 53.

slams that foot down and grounds it, the odds are that his leg is going to buckle in. The most natural reaction is to try and stiffen up and resist your moving his leg in. Dumb move, namely because unless he connects it to the earth so he can use his body weight to counter yours, his leg muscles just aren't going to be up to the task. Try it; stand on one foot and have someone push your leg in an inverse kind of direction.

Hopefully by this time there's a little light bulb going off in the back of your head. Sort of a vague sense of, "Hmmm, this is somehow important." Stop and look at any drop step that I've told you about and check out how an inversion impact could work against you! That's part of the reason why I told you to stomp. A stomp roots you down right quick and is like trying to deflect a train. Trying to do an inversion move against an oak tree that's suddenly rooted there ain't real easy. Part of getting your ass rooted down fast is keeping these same nasty things I'm telling you to do from happening to you.

Taking Away His Support

For you real rocket scientists, you might have also noticed that I mentioned the two escapes out of this move not one paragraph back. Remember one of Uncle Animal's training tips: spend half your time studying how to do a move and the other half studying how to fuck it up! That way when someone is so tacky as to try it on you, you will have a rude surprise waiting for them. It also gets you accustomed to what it feels like when something goes wrong so you don't continue with it and end up putting your dick in the microwave.

Blowing the guy's foot out from under him is one way of doing it. To tell you the truth, the more experienced your opponent is, the less likely it is to work effectively. By definition (at least my definition), the more experienced a guy is, the more likely he is to have encountered something like this before. If he doesn't know the exact counter to the specific move you're doing, the odds are he's encountered something close enough that something else he does will work. This, by the way, is why martial arts instructors look so impressive to new students; a trick the student would have never thought of by himself is old hat to the instructor. Usually the instructor shows why the move wouldn't work on him (therefore the supposed attacker he's training you to fight off) and why "his" system is the best, because it always works against the aforementioned attack.

There are three basic flaws with this assumption. First, the odds are that any attacker is not going to be as well-trained as he is; therefore, there is a damn good chance that it *would* work on the asshole, especially if the dude is drunk. Second, I'll lay you dollars to donuts he's not showing you the simple counter to that move that would put him or any other practitioner of his style on their ass. Finally, you ain't him, he ain't your attacker, and it's your skill level against an attacker that counts. Why spend years training to fight experienced tournament fighters when that isn't what you're going to be running into in the real world? A drunk attacks like a drunk, not a sports fighter or a trained martial artist! A head-down, arms-wide drunken charge is a bitch to defend against. A street fighter fights like a street fighter, and a barroom brawler is just that. A manic explosion could mean anything from flying furniture to a wrestling match between him and ten of your team to him running around wildly waving a meat cleaver. Do any of those sound like anything you've ever seen in the ring?[1]

When some whipdick challenges you with the "why don't you get in the ring" question, do what I do—challenge them right back to face off drunks, manics, and felons every day for a year or two and see if they can live through that. Nothing like a drug freakout with a piece of pipe to keep you humble.

Okay, I'll get off my soapbox now. Anyway, like I said, the more experienced the dude is, the more likely he is to counter the move by simply putting his foot down fast. You run this risk even if you're motherin' fast. On the other hand, if the dude is drunk or otherwise impaired, it often works just peechee keeno. Above all, your timing is important. Snake in on the dude before he can get his weight onto that foot.

Now let's look at another one of my personal favs.[2] That is the foot hook. Instead of trying to push the dude's foot inward at a critical time, you hook your foot around his ankle and drag it outward. This move is harder to perfect, but once perfected it is a total bitch to defend against. It will drop most people. Even trained martial artists bite the dirt on this one because there aren't that many hard styles that include this sort of stuff until you get into the eighth or ninth dan level.

Depending on how effective and nasty you are with this kind of move determines how much damage you inflict. You can do everything from just knocking the guy onto his ass to causing him to fall in the splits and rip ligaments and muscles from asshole to kneecap to having him fall head first into the asphalt and die with a cracked skull. Know how much money you have available to pay your lawyer and decide on which one you want to do.

Taking Away His Support

Before we go on with the heel hook, let's look at the related move (also one of my favorites) that is this same principle applied to would-be Von Dumbs with those fancy kicks. Simply catch and lift any kick that a moron throws at you above waist level. I cannot tell you how many times I've seen people knocked onto their asses as a direct result of high kicks. I'm talking on the street, I'm talking in the ring, I'm talking on the mat. What's scarier is how many times people end up on their ass just by sheer accident!

Okay here it is. Laughing boy throws a kick at you. All you gotta do is catch it. Yeah, right.

Don't worry, I ain't going to leave you hanging. You can do it one of three ways. One is to block the kick and try to grab it immediately. If the guy is stupid enough not to get out as fast as he went in, this works. If he's got the reflexes of a rattler or if he's trained, you might not get a chance.

Number two, you can open your defenses and just let the kick land. Once he's inside your guard you spring the trap shut. Hurts like a bitch, but it's probably the most reliable way to guarantee you're going to get a hold of his leg. The impact is going to slow him down, and you can muckle onto him like a lobster with an attitude.

Number three, however, is what I recommend, which is sort of a blend of the first two combined with a step/pivot, better known as rolling with the punch. In whichever direction the kick is headed, you go that way too for a step, as in Figure 54. Not only does this reduce the impact that you're going to take, but by pivoting with the force you deflect more of it. By throwing up your hands and letting him crash his way through a few barriers, you further slow down his attack and bleed off energy. Finally, by moving out of the blow's target range, you're escaping the apex of its force, as most blows are designed to deliver most of their energy at a certain location. It's like a depth charge set to go off at a certain depth; if you change depths you're going to avoid the worst of it. If he tries to

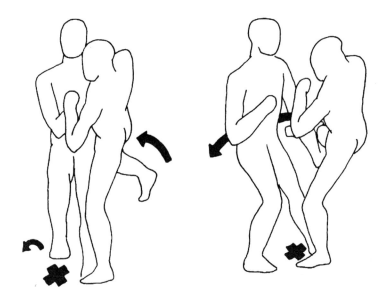

Figure 54. Rolling with a kick.

follow you after that point, he's rapidly going to lose even more clout. Your body is going to absorb the remaining energy and stop the guy's kick.

All of this should have given you time to grab that fucker's foot. From this point you can do one of three things: 1) step back quickly, 2) step forward quickly, or 3) lift (Figure 55). That's it. Well, okay, maybe you should jam his leg first so he can't bend his knee or anything like that, but that's just a matter of putting your hand on his knee. Come to think of it, a corkscrew is kind of fun too.

The first two are the fastest, the third is probably the most spectacular, while the fourth is probably the most bulletproof and the nastiest fall. With the leg lift, you risk taking an extra punch or two before the guy goes down. Also, if he is a martial artist he could be limber enough to make it difficult. On the other hand, that step forward can bowl him over, and the back step can either get him hopping after you or falling into the splits. Like I've said, the

Taking Away His Support

141

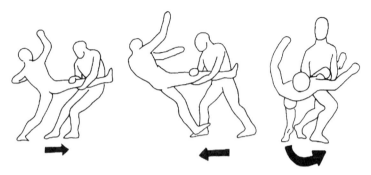

Figure 55.

trick to both of these is to do them quickly. If the guy has a chance to hop around to keep his balance, he will.

Each and every one of these moves is stone-cold illegal in the ring. However, one night when you have nothing better to do, watch a karate tournament on the boob tube and check out how many times someone goes down because something happened while he was attempting a kick. You'll see these basics as the root of most of the falls. This is why I'm not a big fan of high kicking.

Now back to heel hooks. The reason they're called heel hooks is because they're best done from behind the guy's heel. The reason for this is that it is easier to blow the guy's heel out this way than it is from the front. Observe Figure 56 and see what happens when you push against the L of the foot from different directions.

Notice with the first two illustrations that the normal shape of the foot drives the ball of it into the ground if you

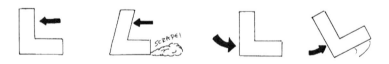

Figure 56.

try to push and lift. This makes it impractical to try and hook someone's foot out from the front. It can be done, but only if the guy's foot is placed really far out from underneath him or you are coming in from the side (like off his shoulder) and you throw something extra in like a hand on his head.

Let's go back a second to subjects I mentioned earlier, eversion and inversion. As I said, a kick against the foot in an inverse direction is a real good thing, while a kick in the other direction is a risky and not real reliable proposition. With a heel hook, however, it's the exact opposite—eversion is good, while an inverse hook is *mezzo mezzo* at best (Figure 57). While it is possible to do an inverse hook on the guy, you end up with the same problems as with an eversional kick: you're likely to run out of leg before it's effective, and if and when the guy falls, you're leg is likely to be under him. Like I said, possible but risky, especially if the guy is in a wide stance.

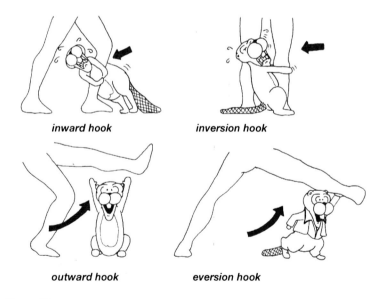

inward hook

inversion hook

outward hook

eversion hook

Figure 57.

Taking Away His Support

Now this doesn't mean that you shouldn't heel hook the guy from any direction you possibly can. What it means is once you hook him, you have a couple of options. Some work better under certain circumstances than others. As we proceed, you're going to find out what is the best option for whatever circumstance you find yourself in.

The best heel hooks pull the guy's foot out from under him. The best way to do that is to both pull and lift (Figure 58). Not only is this action more along the way the guy's leg works naturally (try swinging your leg in any direction— eventually it will go up), but it makes it harder to get out of. The only escape from a heel hook is "up," but that isn't obvious the first time you meet up with one.

Once you're free of his interference, you need to compensate for the damage that he's done to your balance and get your foot back down fast enough to keep you from falling on your ass. Unless you're Jackie Chan and can do impressive feats of balance on only one foot, you'll have less than 2 seconds to identify the danger, escape, reposition your foot so it's past his, and then get it back down in time to save your balance. This task is made more difficult by the fact that the guy is going to be fighting your escape all the way.

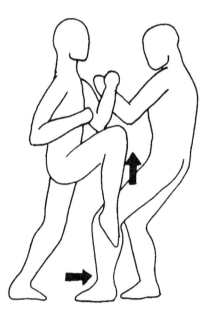

Now that you know how to escape them and mess them up, let's take another look at the best way to do the lowly heel hook. The best source

Figure 58.

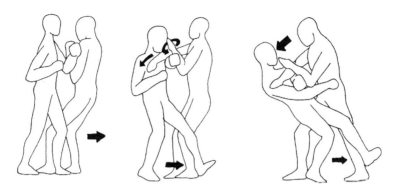

Figure 59. The heel hook.

of power for heel hooks is in your hips. That means when you've hooked the dude, don't try to use just your leg muscles—throw your hips into a pivot and drag your leg with you. In simple terms, step back. Your hook, powered by your body's mass pivoting backward, does wonders for messing up his footwork (Figure 59).

The other type of heel hook calls for a greater control of balance on your part. This is a more advanced technique and requires that you practice it a whole lot before you go out and try it in a live-fire situation. In this one you hook the guy's foot with yours and then basically try to scratch the back of your thigh with your heel (Figure 60). This is where all that Hacky Sack playing is really going to pay off. Of all the heel hooks and impacts, this is one of the hardest to escape from. Of course, you have to have good enough balance not to fall on your ass when you do it.

There are four things I seriously recommend you do when you practice these moves.

Number one: *warn your partner!* Don't just spring these moves on him! They are brutally effective, and unless you both know what you're doing, you can end up hurting someone you don't mean to hurt.

Taking Away His Support

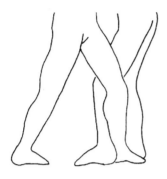
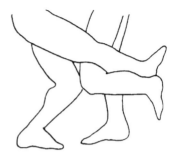

Figure 60.

Number two: during practice, don't take these past the point of falling. Take it right up to the edge and stop. Not only will it keep your partner and you from ripping open at the asshole, but it will keep both of you from taking a header.

The third thing is, any time you do this kind of move on a practice partner, grab him. Encourage him to grab you too. This will help keep both of you from going over.

The fourth thing you both need to do is practice falling and rolling. The amount of damage that you can avoid by knowing how to tuck and roll is immense.

Got all that? Alright, it's time to get back on track. (Sorry guys, sometimes my train of thought makes the U.S. Post Office seem organized.) Anyway, the third way to take someone's support away is by snagging his feet up. Once you've got his feet tied up, you make him move.

Probably one of the more fun dirty tricks I learned when I was a snot-nosed brat was this: as you're coming in swinging on someone, step on his foot. It physically slows him down, and he's going to try to muscle his way out from underneath your weight. While he's trying to squirm out, you're laying in some serious licks upside his head. (If, however, he knows about the hip pivot, he's going to drag your ass into exactly the kind of splits situation we were just talking about, so be careful.)

A Professional's Guide to Ending Violence Quickly

Most people are totally dumbfounded for a second when something as simple and natural as taking a step is interfered with. I'm talking blank looks of confusion and often freezing in shock! Face it, 99.9 percent of your life, when you try to take a step, it works. In fact, it is such an assumed action that once you've reached your second birthday you generally quit thinking about it. It's autopilot stuff. Even a drunk pays more attention to aiming toward the middle of the three doors he's seeing than actually walking!

It's messing up that basic process that suckers in more people than you can shake a stick at. A little while ago, Richard (he of my knife video fame) and I ran into each other. He'd been teaching pentjak silat up in Santa Cruz and had a new list of nasty tricks. Naturally, I wanted to know them.

We faced off. The next thing I knew, this 6′3″ dude had thrown himself down to the ground and pretzeled his ass all around my feet. My initial reaction of "what the fuck are you doing?" was quickly replaced with the realization that my feet weren't going anywhere, but the rest of me was traveling outside the cone of my balance. Where did that body check come from? Oops.

He did about three more "diving to the ground" moves, which on the surface looked like suicide, but they were all nasty trippers. They were designed to send someone crashing to the ground in the most unpleasant ways. Basically, the only way out was to sprout wings and hope for the best.

What makes snagging someone's support so vicious is it gives you complete control as to when you're going to let go of it so he can do something about his falling. Those funky floor moves of Richard's made it impossible to twist, tuck, and roll to handle the fall without breaking your ankles. Great choice—busted ankles or a full-force slam into the ground. No thank you. If you have access to a mat, go out and do a few tucks and rolls and watch your feet. Man, do they move a lot. (By the way, for those clever ones who'd like to go out and experiment, I don't recommend trying to fall without moving your feet, as it's a good way to get hurt.)

If you want to invest a few years in studying some of the nastiest techniques along these lines, go find a real pendakar who's at least 40 years old. For those of you who don't have that kind of school nearby, judo and jujutsu will serve in a pinch. In the meantime, however, let's look at some of the basics here.

In a nutshell, snagging basically means locking someone's foot/feet up and then getting them outside their cone of balance. Push or pull, it doesn't matter. After that, gravity does the work for you. Figure 61 sums it up nicely.

Generally, there are two ways to get him outside of his cone of balance: let him do it himself or push him. Pretty simple, eh?

The first one is what judo claims to be all about in using the guy's force against him. He throws a punch, you dodge, catch it, and do a step pivot and drag the guy forward. In the process you leave a leg out there for him to

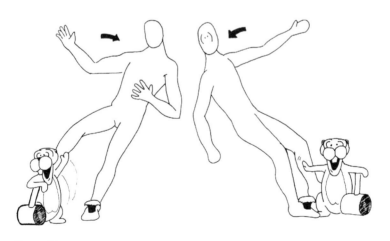

Figure 61.

trip over. Suddenly his body is moving forward and his feet are way behind. Guess who's going to meet Mother Earth in a second?

Quick, easy, and effective . . . maybe. The fundamental problem I have with this sort of situation is that the guy *has* to commit his body weight to a punch. Granted, this is going to qualify about 85 percent of everyone you're going to run into out there. I'll go into the Murphy's Law problems with it in the next chapter.[3]

Realistically, there are many a time when it's not in your best interest to let the guy get off the first shot. If you wait until he gets his body weight in motion so you can use it against him, the chances of something going wrong increase. That means instead of it being a simple throw, it can easily turn into a furball (as in two cats fighting). When this happens, you're going to get hurt. With the high HIV infection rate among drug addicts, convicts, and mental patients, the idea of rolling around on the ground with a guy and both of you bleeding really loses its appeal.[4]

It's also kind of a drag waiting around for the other guy to move perfectly for you to zap him instead of waiting for him to put himself into a position where you can use his weight against him, so you might want to consider doing it to him.[5] The most basic move along these lines is, as I said, simply to step on his feet and shove him. Do it fast enough and he is going to go over like a tree. Do it too slow and he's going to recover. Then again, if he's drunk you may not need to be that fast.

Obviously a drop step and what would be an AI strike to his chest works best for this move. From the front you're going against his stance integrity. From the side (with his feet close together), step on his back foot before you shove. The problem with this kind of move is, unless the dude hits something on the way down, there's nothing to interrupt his attitude. In other words, he's just going to be pissed that he got pushed over. Not a good way to stop a fight from happening (unless you kick him in the face as he tries to get up).

Taking Away His Support

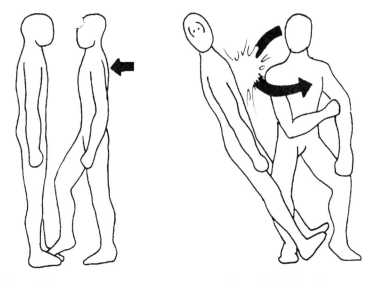

Figure 62.   Note: the heel hook

So let's take it to the next level—you doing a heel hook and pivot. Same thing—snag his feet and shove him out of his cone of balance (Figure 62).

In a pinch you can just use your shoulder/hip to slam into the guy, but the more traditional version is when you extend your arm across his chest and as you sweep him off his feet, you bend forward, thereby directing him to the ground. Not only have I used both, but I've also used hands and elbows backed by a pivot to get the guy going.

As you may have guessed, you can combine your drop step and AI into this one move. Since, as I told you earlier, your feet need to start moving first, by the time your blow lands you've already positioned your foot to snag the guy up. Believe me, an open palm strike to the face followed by slamming him into the ground will change his attitude.

As I've described it, I would give this basic snag about a 75 percent efficiency rate. Let's increase those odds. Remember, as he's going over he's going to try to grab you, so

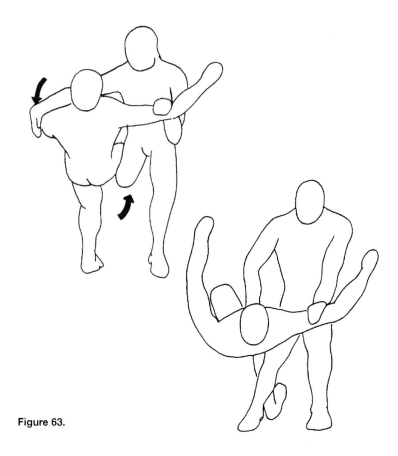

Figure 63.

keep that other hand available for brushing him off. Not only will this keep him from taking your ass over with him, but if you don't go over, it will keep him from hanging on to you and not going himself. (I've had it happen!)

Another thing that will make this more effective is, after you've kept your footing when he ran into you, if he's tottering on the edge of the point of no return, lift your hooking leg backward (Figure 63). Since he's hooked onto that leg, this action will change his balance and cause him to go over. The arm across his chest makes it more effective but also increases the chance that the guy will glom onto it and

Taking Away His Support

drag you over too. (By the way, the proper Japanese judo term for this move is *usoto gari*.) My personal preference is a palm strike to the dude's chest (as shown in the second drawing in Figure 63) because I can straighten my arm to push him down without bending over too far myself, but do what you feel most comfortable with.

Now, the things that Richard was showing me were absolute horror stories because they snagged up both feet before shoving you into the atmosphere. Whether by using hands or feet, they grabbed both of my legs and made it impossible to fall well. I have to tell you right here and now that the one-foot hook is less reliable than snagging up both of the guy's feet. But there is a catch.

The tradeoff for being less reliable is that one-foot snags are faster. Two-leg snags are generally slower and more complicated, but they are much more bulletproof once you get the guy into them. That's the problem—unless you're real good, it can take too long to get into that position. While you're moving into that position, you're vulnerable. I think the problem is obvious.

My recommendation is to get the basic snags down pat. Make them your bread and butter moves. Save other more complicated moves for special occasions.

Again, let me harp on the fact that *Floor Fighting* is the companion book to this one. A lot of other relevant information is touched upon in it for those times when, despite your best efforts, Murphy rears up and bites you on the ass.

ENDNOTES

1. By the way, until they're fighting on concrete with two or three against one, surrounded by tables and chairs and boxed in by either an iron fence or brick wall, the "ultimate fighting" contests ain't really either. Granted it's the closest I've ever seen, but it ain't there yet. They're fighting for money and glory; you're fighting for your life.

2. Funny, most people have favorite TV shows; I have favorite ways to maul people. Sheesh.

3. If you don't want to go to the ground with the guy, just kicking a running suspect's back foot into his other leg is loads of laughs. It is the same principle—his feet are snagged up, and his motion carries him out of the cone of balance. He can slide up to 10 feet on a slick floor or loose gravel.

4. I highly recommend you read *Floor Fighting* if you are in a profession where you're likely to end up on the ground with someone.

5. Sun Tzu said, "It follows that those who are skilled in war can make themselves invincible, but they can't cause an enemy to be certainly vulnerable."

   Mei Yao Ch'en replied, "That which depends on me I can do; that which depends on the enemy cannot be certain."

   Animal sez, "Be careful about spending too much time learning moves that depend on your opponent either stepping on his dick or moving a certain way."

CHAPTER 9

Slaving

"One must take advantage of the situation exactly as if he were setting a ball in motion on a steep slope. The force applied is minute but the results are enormous."
—Chan Yu

There are loads of people who are more qualified to speak on this subject than yours truly. As a matter of fact, anyone who's ever studied aikido, jujutsu, or judo will have volumes more things to say about this topic. To this library of literature, then, I just add one chapter, which will hopefully help you decipher the 18 layers of bullshit you're going to encounter in that library.

Once again, "slaving" means making him susceptible to your motion. Whether it's to your body weight or until his tendons run out of slack, he's going with you. Generally, this occurs until gravity takes control of him or until he runs into a wall.

The simplest form of getting him to endure the effects of gravity/motion is just to tackle the fuck. (Yes, the same move mentioned in Chapter 7. I told you there was overlap in these three basics.) You're best bet is to hit him perpendicular to his line of stance integrity. And, as any football coach will tell you, the lower the better. Not real sophisticated, but it works. Also, as I've said before, this simple little move can work on you just as easily, so be careful.

What I've been talking about up to this point is what happens if you affect the guy's balance from point-blank range. That means shoulder slams, hip pivots, CG slaps, and other close work. I personally have found that going to the source of the guy's balance is the most effective way to get him to lose it.

I will be the first to admit that my fondness for this particular form is mostly based on my size. Ever since I had a 6'5", 300-pound gorilla pluck me off the back of a truck by my belt and dangle me in the air for a few seconds, I knew that I didn't want to stay in the effective range of these kind of guys. For a smaller fighter it is imperative that you get inside a bigger opponent's effective range and then keep on moving. In this sort of situation his longer limbs get in his way while you're zipping around like Mr. Busy Beaver.

Also, 160 pounds slamming into his center of gravity *will* affect him no matter how big he is, while the same may not be true about that same mass tugging on his arm, especially if he isn't out of balance while moving. If the guy is that much bigger than me, I definitely don't want to take the chance of his first attack even being partially successful. Hard to judo fu someone who just reaches out and swats you like a bug.

There are other schools of thought that spend a good deal of time affecting the guy's center from way out in the boonies. If you are close to the same size or bigger than your opponent, then this sort of thing works just fine. So let's take a look at a few of them.[1]

People often classify judo, jujutsu, and aikido together in the same field. Not exactly correct, as they do have different focuses. Although there is much overlapping, an extreme simplification (and I apologize for such a gross simplification) is that judo throws are done from point-blank range (wrestling), jujutsu involves joint locks and twists that cause the guy to either throw himself onto the ground or get a broken arm, and aikido is grabbing the guy's head or arm and dragging him onto his face by using both his momentum and your body weight.

Arguing which one is better is like arguing whether getting laid is better than getting a blow job. Arguing which one is the "ultimate" is even more stupid, as variety is the spice of life. You'll find yourself in situations where each one has its strong points and weak points. I highly recommend you become passingly familiar with all three arts.

The most fundamental move for this sort of fighting is to lock your mass onto his in such a way that it's going to affect him in the negative. It's that added weight/motion you slap onto him that blows him out of the water. By this time the application of the drop step and pivot should be second nature to you (I hope). Yet often in this realm it is applied not in the push but rather the pull.

In other words, instead of slamming into the guy, you pull him. Thing is, you've already set up the physics for this motion with the drop step. Take a look back at Figure 8. Remember, the action that pushes one side of your body forward also pulls the other side backward. Also Sherman, while we're setting the Way Back Machine, let's look at part D of Figure 17 from the same chapter. It's what you do when you avoid a punch. Hell, while we're at it, take it back to Figure 5, the picture of what happens once a force has been delivered. That's what you can use after you've delivered your AI to the chump. Pay close attention to these three, as herein lies most of the secret of making sure the dude flies onto his head.

In any situation, your drop step or corkscrew is what gives the action *cajones*; i.e., this is what adds your weight/motion onto his. It's not just using his body weight/motion against him, nor you throwing all of your weight around. The absolute best combo is a blending of the two. Watch practitioners of the "throwing" arts closely and see how familiar these graceful steps they're doing are to you now. The reason it looks so effortless is because the dude's doing a controlled fall!

It may look like the guy isn't exerting any force, but that's only because he isn't meeting the dude head on. His entire moving body mass is behind that grip he's got on his opponent. And that, my friend, is a shitload of energy going on, no matter how graceful and easy it looks. With all that energy, it's no wonder that you can grab someone and flip him into the dirt. If the dude is off balance to start with, it's going to be all that much easier.

Generally, the most common way of slaving someone to your mass/motion is by grabbing his neck, his shoulder, or his arm and pulling. What makes the first two work is that there really isn't that much slack to absorb your force in the guy's head and shoulders. If done right, there ain't that much slack in his arm either.

That "done right" bit is really important. For example, most of the arm grabs along these lines are done in such a way that either locks the arm into a fixed position (all them wrist/arm lock thingies) or grabbing the arm at the extent of his reach. (Face it, the guy's arm is only so long.) In either

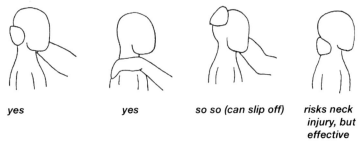

yes   yes   so so (can slip off)   risks neck injury, but effective

Figure 64. Grabbing the head, shoulder, or neck.

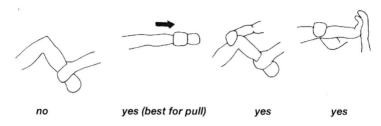

no   yes (best for pull)   yes   yes

Figure 65. Grabbing the arm.

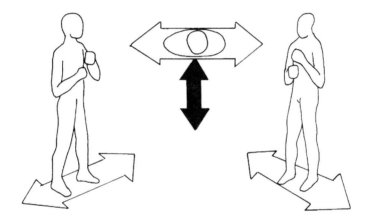

Figure 66.

case, the extra slack is removed, hence any absorption of pressure due to flexibility.

What you have created in all of these circumstances is a direct link to the guy's vertical axis (his centerline). Any force applied to this link will have a direct effect on him. In other words, you've "slaved" him. All that remains now is for you to push or pull in the right direction.

One thing that makes all of this ever so much easier is to push/pull in a direction perpendicular to his stance integrity as often as possible. He's less likely to be able to muster up any resistance if he's already falling over. On the other hand, if you try and fight his stance integrity, it's going to be a hassle and probably not be very effective. Fighting against his stance integrity generally will slow you down and increase the odds of something going wrong. However, by going perpendicular to this line, you encounter less resistance. No matter how he places his feet he's going to have this weakness inherent in his stance.

The forward pull (Figure 67) is really favored by many people. Aside from the fact that it will cause the dude to land face down, it also has the added advantage of working in a direction that we normally bend anyway. And you know what that means. Yep, he goes over easier.

I think by now it would be obvious that you pull down as well as forward. It's your falling, spinning body mass that's moving him, so you might as well drag him in the direction you're heading instead of just forward. I'd also like to point out that this is a real popular move among wing chun fighters, where the neck grab is delivered either with the same hand that just delivered the AI or with the other hand immediately after you've rung his chimes. Oh yeah, if your foot just happens to get in the way of his, this trick works much better (to say nothing about a CG slap).

The thing that makes this more effective is the steeper your downward pull, the less likely the guy is going to be able to regain his feet. You pull too much forward and not

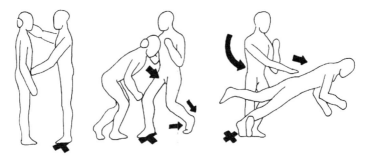

Figure 67. The forward pull.

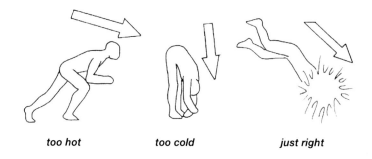

| too hot | too cold | just right |

Figure 68. Angles of pull.

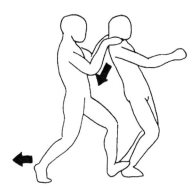

Figure 69. Backward pull.

enough down and he ends up running around you. If there isn't a handy wall around, eventually he can regain his composure and break your nose for what you did. If you pull too close to straight down you end up fighting those same muscles that he uses to fight gravity. Not real effective. It's a happy marriage between forward and down that takes the guy to the ground. (See Figure 68 if this doesn't make any sense to you.) This is why either a corkscrew step or just buckling your knees combined with a forward/ downward jerk usually does the trick.

As you may have guessed, the same move can be applied toward the rear (Figure 69). Like its forward cousin, a well-placed foot in his way can supply you with hours of amusement.

By now it should be obvious to you what slipping a punch and muckling onto the dude's arm while doing a drop step pivot can do to him. You're not contesting his energy; all you're doing is dragging him forward with yours. Remember, you're taking away his control of his own energy. Nine times out of ten the guy is going to be off balance when he punches anyway, so your added energy and weight is going to take him outside his funnel of balance, as in Figure 70.

This kind of move really does work wonderfully well against drunks, amateurs, and inexperienced fighters. Under these circumstances, size really doesn't matter, since the dude has done most of the work for you regarding getting him near the point of no return. This, by the way, is exactly where you end up seeing a little master throwing around six gorillas.

Being as I really do have a habit of pissing on the martial arts PR machine, let me tell you right here and now that against a trained fighter or someone who doesn't commit his body weight to a punch, a thundering herd of these kinds of moves are as effective as a fart against a tornado. Waiting for such a guy to leave an opening that you can exploit is an invite to having your face rearranged. Keep this in mind as you size the guy up.

A trained fighter will move in on you in balance, and he can deliver body weight blows without going off balance. If

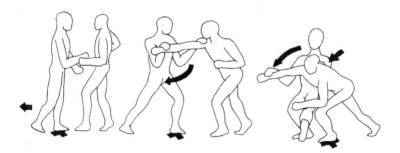

Figure 70.

he's real good he can stop his forward motion, dig in, and brace against your pull. I've seen more than one aikidoist get this surprised look on his face when the dude "grounds" out on him. It's usually followed by an expression of extreme pain when the dude decides to move in that direction anyway, but it's heralded by a stepping punch.

The other time that you might discover that it's not all beer and skittles is against a boxer. The guy may decide to sit back and tenderize your face with a few setups and rattler punches before he moves in with a Nighty Nite Bunny Rabbit blow. He'll dance around and chip away at you, not ever giving you the opportunity to use his own weight against him. Unless you can trap him with the geography and close with him, he's not going to commit until he's ready . . . and when he's ready, it's going to be with something nasty. This is another reason why you want to end it quick. God help you if a boxer gets up to speed. In fact, I'm more leery about mixing it up with a so-so boxer than nearly 95 percent of competent but traditionally trained martial artists.

Against anything that even looks like the situations I've just described, your best bet is to go for one of the other two options: blow his balance or go after his support instead of trying to flip him. Even the professionals do this. Watch how many times the Gracies go after these rather than a fancy dan move to toss the guy when they're up against someone who's a trained fighter. The problem about this is you're going to have to take a few shots getting into position.[2]

While it's easier to take someone over forward or backward, every now and then you gotta take the guy over to the side. There are two ways to do this: you on the side or you in the front.

From the side, make sure the dude isn't in too wide of a stance, grab him either by the neck or at the elbow, and jerk him over. Naturally, this is powered by a backwards drop step (Figure 71). If that isn't possible, a pivot can sometimes work.

Slaving

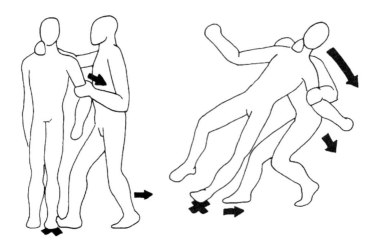

Figure 71. The side drag.

You can either start this move with your foot braced against his ankle or supply one in his path to keep him from getting his foot out there to save him in time. Then again, with most drunks they can't get their feet out there in time anyway. If during an arm grab it doesn't look like it's going to do the job, slap on a neck grab and finish his descent. By the way, don't forget to step out of the way. It's really embarrassing when the dude you just took down plows into you and you both go ass over tea kettle.

This is one of the few moves that can work even if the guy is in a wide stance, as it takes his head out of his funnel of balance if you do it fast enough. If you don't do it fast enough, he is going to lock up his muscles and you're going to be pushing against a rock.

Now as odd as it may sound, every now and then you're going to have to take a guy over sideways from the front. While generally I don't like doing two-handed grabs on someone from the front (who knows what he's got in his other hand that you may want to defend against), in this particular case it's sort of necessary.

Grab him by either neck or shoulder (preferably the neck) with one hand; the other hand grabs the inside of his elbow on the side he's about to go flying toward. Do this at the base of his biceps so your hand is braced on either his elbow proper or against the bulge of muscles on the end of his forearm.

This placement is real important, as it is what will keep you're hand from slipping off as you apply your body weight. The combination of bone protuberances and muscle mass will allow you to brace your hand against them as you jerk. What you don't want to do is grab the guy's forearm at the thickest part because that's like grabbing onto an icicle and pulling down—you're going to slip down his arm. Even if you miss the exact spot and end up hitting high on his biceps, tighten your grip as you slide down. Eventually you'll reach the place where your hand will jam against him. Once that happens, you're not likely to break free of your own grip when you apply the jerk. By the way, the same thing applies to the first sideward grab I just told you about—grab above the elbow.

One of the first things you need to do once you get into this is straighten your arm in the direction he will soon be

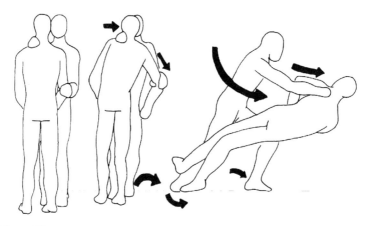

Figure 72.

Slaving

traveling to eat up any slack and establish a direct link to his centerline. Do this as a quick jerk, as it not only eats slack but pulls him off balance. Once you have him tightened up, he's ready for a flying lesson. Now corkscrew down. Unlike normal procedure, in this situation you're going to have to rely on your pivot and arm muscles rather than falling body weight to send the dude flying directly over to the side. So don't forget to go to the gym before you try this.

A simple variation works here if you're not really in the best position to grab his flight-side arm (like he's flapping it around too much to grab it); that is to slap one hand on his neck and the other on the same-side shoulder (Figure 73). Your pivot/drag against his neck will get him started. Once you get moving, shove suddenly with the arm on his shoulder. The push is in the same direction he's going; it adds speed to his trip.

Once, in a moment of drunken "get out of my way," I threw a guy nearly 25 feet off a hillock using this move. I don't know if that's a world record, but I do know that it's an Animal record. The only thing the poor guy did was get in between me and more beer with a smart comment. I just chucked him aside and kept on going toward the keg. I wouldn't have even looked back if it hadn't been for the shocked looks on everyone else's faces.

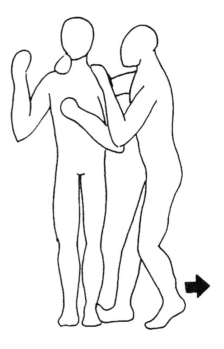

Figure 73.

I would also like to point out that the front version of this move is *great* for buying you distance. If you find yourself in something that is a little more intense than what you planned for, this move can get you enough time to get reorganized, especially if there is more than one of them. It has saved my ass many a time due to the fact that somehow I always seem to throw a guy into at least one of his friends. They both go tumbling over, and I can turn my attention to other things. Also, if you discover that you're suddenly facing a weapon, a handy wall can do all sorts of fun things to the guy's good looks.

Now a more graceful version of this exists where you can do a backward drop step and instead of throwing the guy to the side, you drag him *around* you in a direction that can only be called over your shoulder. (Take your hand and point over your other shoulder. It's that way.) However since every time I've tried to do this move I've ended up kissing a drunk asshole, either I ain't doing it right or it is a highly overrated move. So if you want to learn it, go ask someone else.

A fundamental move in any of these sort of elbow-grabbing moves is to get the guy's arm in the direction you want to throw him either before or as you're starting to apply your body weight (Figure 74). Face it, the upper arm is only so long, but you have to make sure the connection is without slack first. That's why you have to get his arm there first. Of course, you'd be amazed at how many times the guy is nice enough to do it for you.

If you're a lazy fuck like I am, you'll just wait until the guy places his arm in a direction that is perpendicular to his stance integrity and then either push or pull. Oh, didn't I mention that in a pinch you can also create a direct link by trying to push his elbow into his shoulder? It's another one of those "oh shit, I gotta get some room here" moves. Not something that you want to rely on all the time, but it can work.

This brings up another thing that I've seen done but am basically too short to use effectively—shoving someone

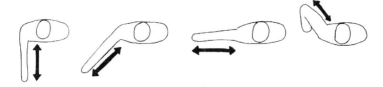

Figure 74. Arm positions for throw.

over by first lifting them up. I've seen a few bouncers move guys toward the door this way. They walk up, grab the guy's elbow when his arm is down, and lift it toward the shoulder, often snaking their arm through (Figure 75). This jams his shoulder and lifts one side of his body off the ground. Then they grab his other shoulder with the other hand and steer him out.

What this does is tilt the guy over and prevent him from moving his other leg to catch himself and resist. The leg he has to move is the only thing keeping him up at the moment. The push gets him moving (mostly running to keep his feet under him) toward the door. I've seen bouncers actually trotting after people, reaching out now and then to shove them just enough so they don't regain their balance. It sort of reminded me of watching a kid with a stick swatting a rolling hoop down the street.

The advantage of this is you can get the guy going toward the door, and thus far you haven't hit him, nor have you thrown him to the ground. If laughing boy comes up swinging, he's the one who took it over the line, at least according to the witnesses. The disadvantage to

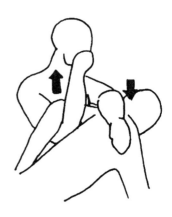

Figure 75.

all of this is, if he regains his feet, he will come up swinging. The times I've seen it used were generally against drunks who were really obnoxious but just shy of the line where you could justify them "slipping." This move generally takes it over the line.

As I said, I never have really been able to use this move, so I can't give you a rundown on its strengths and weaknesses. I've seen it work for bigger guys, but I would have to stand on my tippy toes to make it work for me. As you can guess, it's hard to look butch in that position.

In my book *Floor Fighting* I spent all sorts of time explaining how to mess up attempted joint locks, which is the other way to get someone down to the ground. So I won't bother writing about them here, except to say that I have some reservations about them.

Personally, I consider joint locks to be the height of elegance, grace, and delicacy. However like most art, while I admire them, I often question their application in a hot situation. This is not a matter of *if* you should use them, but *when*.

The root of this issue comes from priorities and limitations put on professionals by those people who aren't out in the field risking their ass, and from the blanket use of the term "control." If controlling a situation is something that you can do all at once, then fine. In this case, however, control means that about six other things fall into line once you find the key component and apply it.

Ah, there go I but for the grace of Murphy . . .

Those who have little experience in real-life adventures like to think that physically controlling someone can be accomplished in one simple act. Slap a wrist lock on the guy and gently take him to the ground without hurting him. However, for those of us who have actually faced the slobbering hordes, we know it isn't all that simple, nor is it likely to be quick. Under these circumstances, that so-called key may not be as applicable to everything that's going on as the Monday morning quarterbacks would think.

When faced by a hairball situation, you have to take that

blanket term of "control" and break it into its component parts. (Could it be that control isn't the most basic issue?) What you have to do is prioritize these components as to which one you will address first. In this sort of situation, we can take a lesson from southern California fire fighters, who, when confronted with the monster brush fires that ravage the area, have a pretty simple set of priorities. While the ultimate goal is control, their priorities are 1) save civilian lives, 2) save homes, and 3) control the fire.

If it were possible to put out a brush fire all at once, then these priorities wouldn't be necessary. And with many of the smaller fires this is possible. The same thing applies to physical violence. The smaller problems you can take care of all at once. However, like brush fires, since it's often no longer small by the time you get there, you have to prioritize as to which issue you're going to handle first.

Many people mistakenly believe that when I say "get the guy to the ground," I'm talking about controlling him. I'm not. I'm just talking about neutralizing the threat. On the ground the guy is much less of a threat to others and me. He's not under control yet, but he's going to have a hard time attacking the person he's pissed at while he's laying face down on the pavement (to say nothing about attacking me). My first priority now and always has been to *neutralize the threat!*

If a situation occurs where you can both neutralize the threat and control him at once, go ahead man! If you can not only get the guy down but do so in a restrained position, lay one on the sucker and pat yourself on the back for a job well done.

With all of my experience, however, I have to say that I have rarely encountered a situation where the guy just naturally stepped into a position where I could lay such a whammy on him. More often than not I had to schlep over and get into a position where I could use such a move. For the most part, all of this was happening before the situation went down. In other words, it was a tense situation, but it wasn't a hot one yet. If and when the dude decided to get froggish, I could lock one onto him, provided he didn't jump in an unexpected manner, at which point it was open season. If it suddenly went hot, God knows how the dude was going to move! Whether I was standing 3 feet away, up close, in a clinch, or on the ground changed from second to second. And nobody could predict which one it was going to be, much less manipulate the guy into position to use a particular move.

Look at all of those qualifiers I just mentioned! You'd be hard pressed to find more "if I could only do this" and "if he'd only do thats" outside a marriage counselor's office. Do you begin to see the problem? Anything that relies on so many ifs is going to be a real shaky thing to bet your dick on! There are just too many situational variations that you're going to be running into not to prioritize if and when it goes down.

Once you have him down to the ground, then a whole shitload of potential problems fall by the wayside. At this point you can seriously consider controlling him. However if you try to "control" him up front, you can actually be trying to come at a general problem from too specific of a direction. (Incidentally, this is one of the main reasons I recommend AIs. They stun the chump long enough for you to put into effect your priorities!)

Once you've taken a hot attack down to the ground, now is the time to drop down and go for specific control. If the guy's lying on the ground, slap a wrist lock on him, put whatever heavy body part you have available on his elbow or neck, slap a nelson on him, or whatever. Just don't let him get back up while he's hostile!

The other problem that I've found about wrist and arm locks come from the realm of physiological effects of alcohol and drugs. Now when you grab a normal person's wrist and twist, he is going to decide quickly that there is way too much pain in a particular area and start doing the mambo to lessen this pain before anything gets twisted off.

Slaving

It's this very reaction that the person using the lock is relying on. However, when you're talking about a drunk, you're talking about someone who is undergoing the physiological effects of a depressant! What do depressants depress? The nervous system!

Why is this important? Because the message to quit fighting before you break something might not get its way through the chump's nervous system before it's too late. While normally the message to quit fighting against your grip would get to him quickly, drugs, alcohol, or extreme emotions can jam his circuits, and he'll resist long after pain should have him throwing himself onto his head.

Now while a drunk can fall down and not necessarily get hurt because he's so relaxed, you are twisting things up in such a way that no matter who it is, if he doesn't cooperate he's going to get hurt. The message of pain will get to the guy eventually, but you may have shattered his wrist before then. If you've ever watched a drunk get taken down, one thing that they always seem to whine about is "you're hurting me!" Even if you're no longer really applying any pressure to the dude's joint, he's still squealing about how much it hurts. Guess what? He's not making it up—the message just got there.

The best way to understand this is to think of it as lag time. He's just now feeling the pain from the takedown! What caused the pain happened a while ago, but the news is just reaching his brain. Keep this lag time in mind before you grab hold of a drunk's joints, because they'll fight you at the wrong time and you'll end up breaking your toys. This is especially important if you have superiors, policies, and lawyers to mess things up.

Again, I would like to restress that arm locks and such are extremely refined and in many cases useful. The best ones, however, are the maneuvers that have been pared down from the flamboyant and elaborate traditional forms and streamlined into quick and useful tools for professionals. Generally, I would recommend that you seriously study

A Professional's Guide to Ending Violence Quickly

the fundamentals I have covered in these last three chapters until you can see them in every situation. And just as important, learn to immediately take the generality, shuffle a few details, and make it fit the specifics of the situation. Then take this knowledge out and fine-tune it by studying the throwing forms. By having the fundamental knowledge under your belt already, you'll not only learn the various throwing forms faster, but you'll be able to tailor their techniques to whatever particular situation you find yourself in.

Also for further understanding, I highly recommend you go out and get C.J. Carracci's video *Practical Hand-to-Hand Combat for the Police Officer*, as it gives an incredibly simple and effective breakdown of a whole lot of these sorts of techniques. As a former training officer, he definitely knows his stuff in this field and can communicate this sort of information in plain English.

Before I finish up, I'd like to briefly touch upon chokeholds. First off, I'm for them. A properly done chokehold can and will knock someone out in about 7 seconds. The entire Rodney King beating could have been avoided if they had been allowed to apply a chokehold on him. Secondly, I'm not going to tell you how to do them because done incorrectly, they can and will kill someone, and the last thing I need is a lawsuit.

Unless you want to face a murder rap, before you even think of slapping a chokehold on someone I would highly recommend you study CPR and a few of the related emergency medical techniques that apply to asphyxiation, especially those related to choking from trauma to the throat.

In addition, if the yo-yo bleeding hearts ever try to take the chokehold away from your local police, I personally ask you to beat feet down to the meeting hall and make pro chokehold noises. Throw in your two cents as a professional who has to face the psychos out there. I would be the first to say that it should be procedure that instead of taking a guy to jail after choking him out, he should go to the hospital instead. Unfortunately, most police procedure manuals beat me to it. Just don't let what happened in Los Angeles happen in your town because someone said the chokehold is inhumane and dangerous. (Hint: it involved a lot of smoke and looting.)

ENDNOTES

1. For those of you who say, "What about Grandmaster So and So? I saw him throw six big guys around," my reply is A) that's him, not you; you're not as well-trained, and B) remember there's that Mic out there named Murphy.

2. For those of you who just went, "Wait a minute, ain't he always saying to *avoid?*" Face it guys, you're gonna get hit sometimes. Realize that I am rabidly against *needless* punishment. If you have to soak up a few to get into position for a move that you know is going to work, then so be it! However I have a real hard-on against getting torn up for a "maybe it'll work if he cooperates" move.

CHAPTER 10

Weapons

"I don't have to be faster than a bullet, just faster than the guy with the gun."

—Amazing Eagle

I was the cooler of a topless bar in Phoenix when my partner and I ran into a problem. I'd stepped out the front door to get a breath of fresh air when a beat-up white land yacht cruised into the back parking lot with two dudes in it.

A few minutes later one guy walked in. Something about the guy had set my bells off, and I'd asked for some ID despite the fact that he was obviously over 21. Surprise, no ID. Now legally I shouldn't have let the guy in, but he started whining and bitching (basically stalling) until he'd called over the off-duty assistant manager (an alcoholic asshole who'd nearly gotten me shot in a previous incident by the road captain of the local biker club). Once again, the AssMan was busy getting drunk. He "vouched" for the dude, and despite the fact that everything told me that the customer was going to be trouble, laughing boy skated in. (Incidentally, for you bouncers, something I learned is every time I was cool and let something like this slide, those were the assholes who gave me problems later. Think about that before you're "cool" with anyone who isn't a regular and has some hinky problem.)

A few minutes later, Dave, my partner for the night, came up and said, "I just saw that guy sneak a beer out the back door." Well surprise, surprise, surprise. I grabbed the four-cell flashlight and we cruised out into the back parking lot. There, with a beer, leaning up against the white land shark, was a tough little *vato* about 18 or 19. Naturally, the beer disappeared behind him onto the trunk of the car. As we were walking up to him, the door opened and who should miraculously come out? Mr. No ID. Such a coincidence.

I walked up and said the normal "How you doing" before asking him where he got the beer. He told me that he'd bought it next door at the Circle K. Okay, lie number one. I told him that he couldn't drink it on the premises. At this time he shifted and I saw the bulge under his shirt.

Click. The little fucker's got a gun . . . new set of rules here. If it goes down, it's going to get ugly.

While he was explaining to me that he was waiting for someone, I casually put my hands in my pockets and looked at him in calm innocence. I took my right hand out of my pocket and pointed my thumb over my shoulder. "Him?" I asked, pointing to Mr. ID with my thumb.

Funny thing was, the kid didn't see the knife in my hand as I pointed. It's normal to have your hand curled up when you point with your thumb, so he wasn't paying attention to the fact that I'd just snaked a weapon into my hand right in front of him. It's amazing what you can get away with if you look casual about doing it.

No ID spoke up. "I don't know this dude."

"Really? Is this your car?"

"Yeah."

"Well, he was leaning up against it."

"Uh, that's okay."

"My partner here saw you bring a beer out here, and there ain't nobody else in the lot."

"I didn't bring no beer out!"

"I saw you bring one out, man," Dave spoke up.

"You calling me a liar?" snarled the *vato* at Dave.

CLICK! Here we go.

"Did he give you the beer?" I snapped coldly.

The kid swung his eyes away from Dave and back to me. Okay Dave, it's one on one now. I got the kid, you cover the other dude.

"No, I bought it."

"Then I ain't calling you a liar, but you still can't drink it here."

Mr. ID started walking around to the driver's side of the car. I wanted to warn Dave, but the kid demanded my attention at that moment. Please, Dave, stop the fucker.

"You called me a liar!"

"I haven't called you anything. But I am telling you you can't drink it here."

I was looking into the kid's flat little reptile eyes. He was ready to attack. Not ready to die, but ready to kill. I let him look back into my eyes. Hopefully he would be able to look deep enough to see where the blood spills on the sidewalk were.

"What do you have in your hand?" Dave suddenly demanded of Mr. ID. Shit, this is getting ugly.

"Nothing," the guy replied.

"Put it down!" Dave roared.

"I ain't got nothin!" the guy protested.

CLICK. Sorry kid. Now if you move you're going to have to die. With your partner armed I can't afford to try to just wound you. C'mon kid, see it! I don't want to have to kill you!

"PUT IT DOWN!" Dave shouted again.

"Alright man." The guy walked over to the tire bumper and laid a black object down.

"Get over there and sit down," Dave snarled

"Let me try and help," Mr. ID said, holding up his hands as he edged around Dave. His energy had changed. Unlike the kid, he earnestly wanted to end the whole thing now.

"You called me a liar," the kid repeated.

Shit, the kid couldn't see past his testosterone. He still wanted a piece of me. All he could see was how he'd been dissed.

"I didn't call you nothing, but I am telling you you have to go."

Mr. ID walked up and touched the kid on the shoulder. "Ernesto, let's go man," he said quietly. (Don't know him, eh?)

"NO! This fucker called me a liar!"

Shit, it's still Code 2 high. Kid, don't go for the gun. Listen to your partner. He's older. He's recognized me for what I am. He knows you're gonna get hurt here. *Listen!* Time to try another approach—one my stepdad had taught me.

"Look, would you accept an apology?" I asked.

"Hey man, he's willing to apologize," Mr. ID said hopefully.

I saw the kid puff up in importance. "Yeah. Apologize."

"There you go," I said. Neat trick, this. You say that and they often go away without realizing that you didn't exactly apologize.

"No man, you apologize!" he responded.

Shit. Now this is getting absurd. The little fucker broke the law, was doing something that would have gotten our asses nailed by the Alcohol Control Board, lied to me from the start, and now thinks that he's the wronged party. Until now I was being professional. Now I was getting pissed.

"If I was wrong I will apologize," I said flatly.

"Apologize."

"He didn't give you that beer?"

"Apologize!"

Man, I'm close to losing my cool. I may just end up killing this little fuck anyway. If he goes for his gun, I can. It would be self-defense. Cool. Go for it, kid.

No, a part of my brain whispers, you're a professional. De-escalate it.

Mr. ID stepped up to me and spoke quietly. "Look man, this is my cousin. When he gets like this there's no reasoning with him. I admit I gave him the beer. We'll leave. Just apologize to him or he won't let it go. Please."

Apologize to this little lying shit? Part of me really wanted the little fuck to go for his gun. Our first moves would happen simultaneously. His first move would be to grab for his weapon while mine would be to slit his throat. That part of me wanted to see the look of shocked surprise on the kid's face as he realized he was dying. Dying because he'd miscalculated who he fucked with. There's a reason why they call me Animal, you little fuck. The blood was pumping again. I took a deep breath.

"If I was wrong, I apologize," I said evenly.

"There you go, Ernesto," Mr. ID said, jumping in. "Let's go man."

"I don't think he means it," the kid said, hanging on.

Mr. ID grabbed his cousin by the shoulder and dragged him toward the car. "Yeah he means it, man. Let's just go! We'll pick up some more beer somewhere else. C'mon man."

ID hustled the kid in the car and, just before he jumped into it, he looked over the roof at me and Dave and said, "Thanks, man."

We watched as the car backed out and drove away. I watched for the kid trying to roll down the window. When they were gone I put my knife back in my pocket.

"Man," Dave said, "I thought you were going to hit him! I would have."

I smiled and walked over and picked up Mr. ID's knife where it had fallen. It was a cheap plastic-handled folder.

"The kid had a gun," I said inspecting the knife. Out of the corner of my eye I saw Dave's face blanch. I handed the knife to him. "You want this?"[1]

Many years earlier . . .

Two female friends of mine had been waiting on my doorstep when I got home from work. I'd closed that night, and it was around midnight when I came rolling in. My first question to them was, "What are you doing here?"

"We were bored," one said. "We decided to come and kidnap you."

Kewl . . . maybe I'll get laid tonight. I love it when opportunity knocks.

"What's there to do around here?" the other one asked.

Hmmm, here's a problem. The only thing open this late at night are bars, pool halls, and restaurants. I just came from a restaurant, so that one's out. That leaves the first two. Unfortunately, the only places that I felt comfortable with were not the kind of places I'd take these two ladies. It was not only because they would feel uncomfortable, but because 1) I wasn't looking for a fight, 2) walking into those places with two women was an invite to trouble, 3) trouble in those places was not a lightweight affair, 4) I didn't have my wrecking crew with me for backup in case something started, and 5) I was being greedy and not about to go someplace where I'd have to share with my friends. On top of all that, I didn't really feel like just hanging out in a bar and drinking. I thought about it for a second before I remembered a pool hall up in Westchester. Friendly little place where the nasties weren't likely to be.

"There's a pool hall I know . . ."

It didn't take long before we were piling out of their car and heading into what I had always considered one of the mellowest pool halls I'd ever been in. (You can get an idea of what I was used to if I considered a pool hall mellow.) In short order we had a table and a pitcher and had settled down to the sort of trivial chatter that seemed so deep at the time. I'd noticed a couple of crusty types a few tables over who were giving me the hairy eyeball, but since they were about 10 years older than me I shrugged them off. All in all we were having a good, relaxed time.

I was leaning over to take a diagonal cross table shot and had paused in that position to exchange banter with the girls. Returning my attention to the table, I was purposely ignoring one of their snide (but accurate) summations of my skills as a pool player when I heard her break off in mid sentence. I looked back over my shoulder to see that one of the crusties had walked right up next to me without me noticing.

"What kind of knife is that?" he asked flatly, referring to a dagger on my belt.

"A Holden dagger," I replied, starting to straighten up. A lot of people mistook it for a Nazi dagger, but it had been around a long time before (as in Viking times long time before) the Goose Stepping Brigade had stuck a backward swastika on it. My time in college was still a few years down the line, but even then I had a thing for history. Still, I'd jammed with a few folks over the knife who thought it meant I was a Nazi despite my dark hair and skin.

Without warning he whipped his right arm and I heard the snap of a Buck knife opening. I saw the flash of stainless steel reflect wickedly over the green felt top of the pool table, and I knew I had better do something fucking quick.

Before he could bring his hand back from his overly wide and dramatic opening, I dropped the pool cue and lunged forward, my left hand grabbing his wrist and my right dropping down somewhere around his belt buckle.

With a loud "DON'T," I heaved him up and slammed him down onto the pool table. Now don't ask me how I managed to do the next few dribbles, as I really don't have any idea except that it's incredible what your adrenal glands can talk you into when someone pulls out a knife. I distinctly remember bouncing the guy about three more times. He dropped the knife on bounce number three, but I must have thrown one or two more in there just to make sure. When he came to a rest, his arm was outstretched over his head and the knife was way down near his chest, so something must have happened that I don't remember, or I just didn't notice. Anyway, he wasn't going anywhere quick.

I whirled around to face his buddy, who had already decided that they had made a serious mistake and was backpedaling with wide eyes and hands held out in front of him. I saw a flash out of the corner of my eye as the bartender came barreling into view holding something down near his leg which I really didn't want to know about.

A few of the regulars came up to support the bartender, and by the time the guy on the table got his marbles back he was surrounded by a group of people who were not on his side. After their blabbering on about how they "weren't going to do anything" and the women and a few other witnesses saying I hadn't done anything to start the trouble, the guys were kicked out the front door.

The bartender looked at me and said, "You didn't start it. You can stay."

I thanked him, but I told him we'd be leaving as soon as I hit the head. You don't hang around places like that after a fight in case the suckers backed up on you with some serious firepower. I swaggered to the bathroom and locked the door. About a second later I was bent over the toilet barfing my guts out from adrenaline and fear. Once I'd washed up, we scurried out the back door to the car and got the hell out of there. So much for a cool place. The women were so freaked out that I didn't get laid, although I seriously needed it after that little episode.

Those two stories exemplify several key aspects of quicktime fighting and weapons. Basically, the two issues are preparedness before it happens and hard-core mauling the sucker if it does go down. In those situations, the quality of mercy isn't strained, it's flat-out torn to shreds. If you're going to stay alive against weapons, you're going to have to think this way.

Even though the first incident didn't end in bloodshed (and thank God it didn't because I couldn't have afforded a lawyer), it still offers a solid comparison between doing it correctly and the most common mistakes when weapons are involved.

First off, when it comes to weapons the need for quicktime goes up to the squared power. If he manages to deploy a weapon you are fucked! I don't care what big-balled yahoo martial arts experts say, if the dude manages to get a weapon out and even generally pointed in your direction, the absolute best you can hope for is damage control!

Face it, all he has to do is one fast move compared to your four fast and heavy ones. Do the math yourself. The odds are in his favor. It's not even a matter of being first! His one move can happen anytime during the process!

What's worse is it doesn't even have to be intentional. A dude who is falling to the ground is going to be flailing around as he goes. If he's empty-handed, all you have to really worry about is him grabbing onto you as he goes. If he's got a knife, his wild flail can cut you from eyeball to asshole just as effectively as a full-on attack! That, by the way, is the number one fuck up of most martial artists when they talk about punching the shit out of someone with a knife.

Want to know a real bitch? Even if you're winning against an armed opponent, you're still in serious risk of losing. Let me ask you a question. If you are getting the shit knocked out of you, what is your first reaction going to be? Yeah, get the fuck out of there! How? Normally, by pulling back and getting your hands in the way as you backpedal! That is a normal human reaction. And if the dude is bare-handed, King Karate is going to mop the floor with him. However, take that same reaction and put a knife in the guy's hand. Suddenly that pull back and wildly waving of hands becomes a whole lot more dangerous. If King Karate charges into that, he's going to need to change his name to King Coleslaw!

I cannot stress upon you enough the need to finish it before he can get his weapon deployed.

What all of this means is your trigger gets moved up, *and the thing that triggers your attack is him going for his weapon!* At least one of your hands goes for his hand going for the weapon, not to take the weapon away but to keep him from even drawing it. It's better if you can keep him from even grabbing the weapon, but failing that, you're there checking his arm to keep him from getting it out. (If it happens to go off and blow his dick off, well that's his problem.) If you can't do that, then keep him from deploying it in your direction.

Think about this. He's going for his weapon so he can attack you while you're attacking him and simultaneously keeping him from drawing his weapon. If the whole thing is going to be over in 3 seconds, guess who isn't going to come out on top? Your best chance for safety relies on getting control of his weapon before he can deploy it effectively.

That's what both stories have in common. In the first one I was waiting for him to go for his weapon as my signal to attack, while in the other, instead of wasting time that I didn't have clawing for my own weapon, I went after him and his before he had a chance to really deploy it!

Few people have undergone the specialized training to be able to handle an attack on their weapon deployment.[2] If they have, you're definitely messing with the wrong folks, and you shouldn't be there in the first place. On the other hand, I recommend you and your buddies do go out and try messing around with it. All of a sudden all those hip turns, hand sweeps, and side steps will really begin to make sense.

Not too long ago I was having a conversation with someone from the "oh shit" league (we're talking a seriously scary kind of guy). I mentioned that I always had a problem with the raging debate over the Weaver vs. Isosceles handgunning stances. They might as well be talking Martian to me. My point was that anytime I'd been on the receiving end of gunfire I was busy hitting the dirt, which is why I now generally prefer the Israeli system for close-quarter work. Face it, I can aim better with the gun held sideways as I'm diving to talk with the ants (anything past 20 feet I rotate back up to normal sights). He, on the other hand, is one of those guys you call in when you have a psycho somewhere in a building with a gun. Not a job I would want to do, namely because they won't let me do it my way.[3] He and I kicked the idea around, and my subconscious gave one of it's famous beer burps that most people would call a realization.

The realization is that once I was older than 18, the only times in my life that someone ever successfully got a shot off or got a blade out on me was when they'd caught me with my dick flapping in the wind. We're talking out-of-the-blue ambush! That guy in the pool hall is a prime example. He walked up to me from my blind side, knife in hand. Where I'm from that's called an ambush. This is why my first reaction is always to neutralize the threat. Depending on how close and how hot that threat is determines exactly how I do it. Those are the only times that I went head-to-head with weapons, basically because I had no choice.

On the other hand, when I knew I was walking into a hot situation where weapons were around but not drawn, then I knew that by focusing on interfering with his going for a weapon, I would have at least a second to piss in the punch bowl. And oh did I. In other words, when I knew it was a hot situation going in, I made sure that I got the drop on the guy either by having my weapon already in my hand (often out of sight, though) or, the second he as much as twitched toward his weapon, by dropping his ass.

IF THE GUY GETS A WEAPON OUT, DO NOT ENGAGE HIM! DROP HIS ASS TO THE GROUND AS SOON AS FUCKING POSSIBLE! This is one of the few cases where you want him to hit the ground as hard as fucking possible. You want him to hit so hard he goes splat! No bouncing here; you want him to act like a dropped watermelon when he hits! If he rips a few tendons, breaks a few bones, and hemorrhages a few vital things, all the better. In fact, this is one of the few times I recommend adding in an extra shove or elbow to his back for him to pick up speed on the way down. The next chapter we'll talk about being humane, but not in this situation.

Incidentally, if the guy has a gun deployed and there are noncombatants around, try to take him over forward instead of backward. It is not unusual for the guy's hand to tighten on the trigger when he impacts. That means a wild bullet. While there is a good chance that the gun may be pointed at you (like generically upward), when the guy goes over backward it often will be pointing elsewhere. That means one of the noncombatants could take a bullet. On the other hand, if the guy is falling forward the bullet is more likely to go into the ground (or at least only hit someone's foot or ankle if it ricochets). Then again, the guy may fall on his gun and shoot himself (which is sort of funny if you think about it; also there's less paperwork). The same thing also applies to taking a guy over with a knife—it's safer for you to take him over forward. Besides, we haven't had a good show of hari kari since Yukio Mishima.[4]

I've said most everything else about weapons elsewhere.[5] Perhaps the most critical thing to remember is the effective range of a weapon. Whatever it is, you don't want to be there. The old saw "rush a gun, run from a knife" best exemplifies this kind of thinking. Once you know why, then you'll understand ranges.

I will leave you with some pretty pictures of what people look like when they're going for weapons . . .

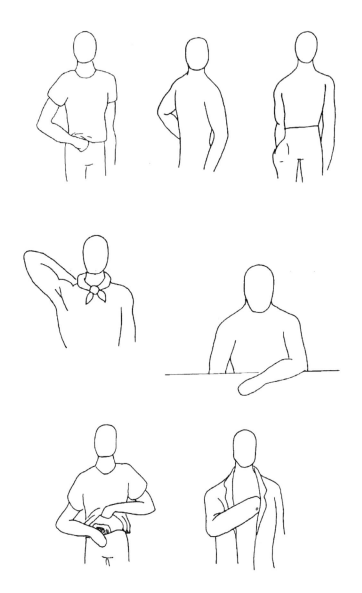

Figure 76.

Weapons

ENDNOTES

1. By the time that story took place I'd already written several books and was the ripe old age of 34. I was the head bouncer because I could keep my cool. Of course I still really did want to maul that SOB.

2. This also applies to most of the throwing arts, which is why I give them such fits. Instead of trying to escape their grip, I attack it. It's sort of like grabbing for a wolverine's tail and discovering he's spun around on you.

3. He said that the powers-that-be frowned on my suggestion of just blowing up the building in those sort of situations. Next to a sniper, it's the most reasonable answer. As long as it's my ass on the line, blowing the building seems reasonable to me. (I keep trying to tell people I'm a coward but nobody believes me.)

4. Mishima was a well-known author in Japan. Aside from being a fanatical follower of bushido, he was also a homosexual. In 1972, he and a group of other militants took over a Japanese Department of Defense building to protest the weakening of Japan's military might. After giving a speech where he urged Japan to rebuild its military (which was mostly drowned out by boos and hisses from the spectators), he went inside and commited seppuku. His lover decapitated him.

5. For detailed information on surviving weapons in general, check out my video *Surviving a Street Knife Fight*. For an overview of the different types of weapons and how to handle them, see my book *Pool Cues, Beer Bottles, and Baseball Bat*s.

CHAPTER 11

Professionals

"Because they stand on a wall and they say, 'Nothing is going to hurt you tonight . . . not on my watch.'"
—*A Few Good Men*

Let's take a quick trip back to the African savanna a million years ago. We have a troupe of primitive humans hanging out chewing on bugs and roots and scratching their fleas. All in all, just another day in prehistoric times. All of a sudden what should pop up but a leopard looking for dinner.

Frantic, 90 percent of the group beats feet, but a small, select band of males do the most absolutely stupid, illogical thing and charge a big, hungry predator.

Why? Hell, they can't tell you. It just seems like the thing to do at the time. Odd thing is, they not only manage to survive the situation, but since they took tools and a willingness to go head-to-head with a leopard, they come out with lunch, a snazzy new set of threads, and some costume jewelry in the form of claws and fangs.

Now rationally you have to admit that charging a hungry leopard does not sound like the height of survival instinct. The smart thing to do would be to haul ass with the rest of the group and do your best to run faster than someone else. That way Slow Foot becomes lunch, not you. There must be something really seriously wrong with anyone stupid enough to buck those kinds of odds and charge Morris on steroids.

Or is there?

Let's take a hard look at doing the "smart thing" and hauling ass. First of all, as males we can generally outrun females, especially as young males. So what would it mean if everyone did the smart thing and ran? Hey, we'd leave the women behind to become tender vittles for Fluffy.

It doesn't take a rocket scientist to figure out that a full-grown female can outrun a small child. Ah, so now we're leaving the kids to deal with Sylvester. Does anyone else begin to see the flaw in this logic by now? Something about species survival?

In the long run, if everyone did the so-called "smart thing," we would have died out as a species a long time ago, and there would have been more than few fat prehistoric kitties. On the other hand, if some young buck is willing to do what looks to be a stupidly macho thing and charge that cat, at worst everyone but him is going to get away. At best there is going to be one less predator out there to threaten the tribe.

The fact that doing this seemingly stupid thing has become ingrained in the male psyche kind of shows that at least one or two of us stayed alive long enough to pass on a heritage of excessive testosterone to the next generation. That means somewhere along the line we also learned a thing or two about handling leopards. Bare hands became rocks, rocks became spears, spears . . . well, you get the picture. Just because we're throwing ourselves at a charging predator doesn't mean we have to abandon all common sense. In case you haven't caught on yet, this is an evolutionary kinda thing.

The reason that I bring up this little story about our ancient past is to give you a slightly different perspective on exactly what we are doing whenever we face off with the predators, criminals, assholes, troublemakers, and flipouts of the world. We're risking our ass so the predators don't get to the rest of the tribe and those who are less able to defend themselves. When trouble starts, we're stepping up and saying, "You gotta get through me before you get to anyone else."

While intellectuals and feminists may bemoan the horrors of macho behavior, what they are doing is ignoring the fact that for nearly two million years that same macho asshole is the one who was keeping them from being the one tangling with lions, tigers, and bears (oh my). Without us watching for trouble and fighting off predators, those folks couldn't live the nice, safe, nonviolent lives they lead.

Now the bad news. In case you haven't noticed, it's not too likely we're going to run into any leopards in the near future. Because of that we have a surplus of young bucks running around with carbonated hormones. Therefore, what we are likely to run into is two million years of evolutionary design bubbling along the synapses of a young man who is also lacking in leopards to fight. In this particular vacuum, guess who he's going to look toward to take this kind of behavior out on? Try other young bucks from another tribe, those of us who step up and say "no" to him, and, often because of some serious dysfunction, generally anyone within arm's reach.

In other words, nearly everyone around him. That very same energy that has kept our species alive for two million years goes amok in a civilized society if we don't find some way to channel it. It isn't a question of "is this energy

Professionals

---

real?" as many intellectuals, feminists, and liberals would like to deny (claiming it is actually a product of psychological/sociological conditioning). It's a matter of, "we have this biological imperative, now what do we do about it?"

Different cultures have come up with different solutions to the problem, whether it be like the ancient Spartans, who designed their entire culture around war, or feudal Japan, American Indians, and ancient Celts, who designated the warrior castes as the elite of society (so the rest of the people could go about their business of surviving), or Confucian China, with it's nearly fanatical allegiance to the family elders and utter subservience by the young, to post feudal Western culture, which considered armies barbaric necessities but a great dumping ground for keeping young bucks out of trouble. Everywhere you go, society comes up with a way to deal with this young male energy. This keeps them from causing too much damage to society in general. Granted you lose a few in the game, but that's just how it works. You can't deal with a level of energy that's willing to take on a leopard without some damage.

Somehow you gotta set it up to keep these loose cannons out of trouble while waiting for leopards and Vikings to show up. Sometimes the best you can do is damage control, where you work their asses off doing hard manual labor and pound a sense of duty into their heads, and any extra energy they have left they spend beating the shit out of each other. Other times you need to put them in an environment where they realize there are bigger dogs around than them, and if they step out of line the old dogs will bite them.

Unfortunately, a thing called the Industrial Revolution sort of put most cultures on their ears. Suddenly the old ways that handled the problem, unjust though they might have been, were thrown out. Much of the hard labor and fighting for survival that took up so much of that energy evaporated along with the pounding a sense of duty to the tribe into the young ones' heads. Now the safety checks were off, but the system was still running.

Unfortunately, along with the bad aspects of that behavior went the controls that kept the young bucks from causing too much damage. That energy is a double-edged sword. It is very easy for it to be twisted and for the possessor, instead of protecting the tribe, to start attacking it and preying on his own. It's just a small step from fighting predators to becoming one.[1] It's no wonder that young males are responsible for most of the crime and violence in this world, because they are the ones who are biologically designed for aggressive behavior. (Actually, make that "we"—I ain't that old yet.)

No amount of argument, persuasive speech, laws, legal mumbo jumbo, psychology, or socialization is going to change this biological fact. You're talking rhetoric vs. an evolutionary survival mechanism.[2] Just as there were a million years ago, there are predators out there today who would attack our tribe. That means somebody has to go out and face those fuckers. The only thing that remains to debate is not that we *have* to do it but *how* we do it.

That's where professionals come in. That's what our job really is—to protect the tribe, sometimes at the cost of our own lives. It's not to run the tribe. It's not to tell the tribe what to do. It's not to make everyone in the tribe exactly like us, nor is it to get our particular clique ahead of all others, but to protect the whole tribe from predators, both internal and external. Whether you're out hunting the predators, keeping them once they've been caught, or standing watch at a hot spot to catch one when they blow, you're there to prevent someone from hurting the tribe.

It's amazing how keeping this in the back of your mind at all times can really shift your perspective. Not only does it help with doing your job, but it helps you to adjust back into the tribe.[3]

Professionals

To tell you the truth, you can't spend all of your time out on the front line. Spending all your time with only those who share the same job is just as damaging and misleading. Much of the misconduct that plagues our profession comes from people who limit themselves to their particular clique. In those situations, the idea of protecting the greater tribe is set behind the idea of protecting one's own clique. Once a clique loses sight of its connection to the greater tribe, then it is very easy for it to become predatory,[4] often while still under the misguided assumption that it's serving its original purpose.

In the same vein, once society loses sight of what it is you are doing and facing, it's real easy for them to forget why it's important to them. In other words, once communication breaks down, everybody goes off into their own agenda and forgets that the whole tribe is made up of other groups, all of which must work together to keep the whole going.[5] You need to constantly be reminded of what exactly you're protecting, and they need to be reminded that the reason they can live like they do is because you're out there keeping the predators at bay. It's not just when you're actively protecting them, but also when you are part of society too. All in all, there's a lot more to this job than most people realize, including those who are doing the job.

You may be wondering why I went off on that soap box speech. If you sort of know why but had never really put it into words yourself, go ahead and use mine. I've found that spiel to be a simple explanation that people who don't have the juice to stand on the wall can understand easily. Since it's more biological than rhetorical, it even makes the most loudmouth "you've been oppressing us" leftist blink in confusion. For those of you who are sitting in the back of the classroom still chewing over the implications of all this, keep on chewing.

Alright, enough philosophy. Let's get back to breaking heads.

One of the biggest bitches about being a professional is the public's belief that by being a professional, you magically become bulletproof, omnipotent, a kung fu master, and somehow better than them. Now while all of this may seem like a real ego boost, in the courtroom it can be a real pain in the ass.

Why? Because if you're all of those things, then you should have been able to "restrain" the PCP freakout with a butcher's knife rather than start pulling the trigger when he was 15 feet away. Both our media and legal system love an underdog. Poor, pitiful so-and-so; he was drunk and busting things up when along came this big, mean professional (who can do all sorts of neat tricks with that big dick of his) who just mercilessly beat up PPSS for no reason whatsoever. Mind you if *you* get hurt, it's all in the line of duty.

Let me tell you right now that your worst enemy is Hollywood. It's not necessarily the media—as big a pack of vultures as they are, they aren't the ones who have set you up. The media may pull the lever, but Hollywood has put the rope around your neck. Every time Steven Seagal or JC Van Damme goes out on the big screen and single-handedly fights off a horde of attackers and only gets artistically placed cuts and scrapes, you get fucked in the public opinion. Why? Because "if he can do it, why can't you?"

Realize that the closest the average person ever gets to real violence is what they see on the screen. Maybe they saw a fight in high school or, oh wow, if it's a guy, maybe he even experienced a fight in high school so long ago.[6] But these people have no idea what real violence is like! It bugs the shit out me when I meet people who think these Hollywood tough-guy martial artists are really as good as their movies make them out to be. No lie, I've encountered more than a few people who thought that! I nearly threw up in the theater when I saw a guy take a 12-gauge shotgun blast at point-blank range to the chest and live! But hey, nobody else in the theater knew how much of a bullshit scene that was.[7] Manly men are supposed to be able to do that . . .

Now let's take a look at a jury of people sitting there with no frame of reference except that sort of nonsense. How sympathetic do you think they're going to be when you say the reason you pulled the trigger was because the dude would have been too hard to take down without you getting mauled? So what if he had a knife and was in the middle of a manic episode? You're a professional!

Tell you what, though. Instead of fighting that perception, let's turn it to our advantage. Let me give you a bit of sage advice. It's something that my first stepfather, a Mexican street fighter from East LA, told me when I was *un pocquito nino*: "Don't hit them in the face; hit them in the body where it doesn't show."

Thanks, dad. Not as much fun as giving me the keys to the car, but much more helpful in the long run.

Let me modify this slightly to be more applicable to the problems we face as professionals: "People see, remember, and are less likely to forgive head shots."

I don't know what it is, but people have a knee-jerk reaction to head shots. If you walk up and slam a guy in the gut with a flashlight, people can and will forgive it faster than if you walk up and lay it upside his head. Even if the head shot is less powerful, people equate it with trying to kill the guy.[8]

There is the belief that, as a professional, you shouldn't have to use head shots. This is unfair and uncool, since laughing boy has no such restrictions, but that's the way it is. In fact, as a pro, just assume that head shots are verboten.

If you play your cards right, though, you can do all sorts of effective shit that people don't even have a clue about and come out smelling like roses. As long as you do certain things to protect the guy's head, you can say you were just trying to control him.

"Why didn't you do anything to catch him?" asks the prosecutor.

(Ignoring the fact that you were the one who actually blew the asshole's balance and caused him to fall.) "Well, sir, once he lost his balance, I knew that I couldn't catch him in time, so instead what I did was focus on keeping his head from slamming into the concrete, which I knew could have been fatal."

Oddly enough, you told the truth. You did grab his head to keep it from slamming into the ground. All of a sudden you're not a bad guy, you're a hero who was trying to save this guy's life. Hey, you're also a real pro who was working to keep something nasty from happening, even though you had to physically restrain the guy.

Notice at no time was the fact mentioned that you wanted everything *except* his head to slam into the ground at full speed? The only thing that grabbing the guy's head does is keep it from whip-cracking onto the concrete when he hits. It doesn't slow his body mass down. He's still hitting hard enough to knock the shit out of him (and maybe break something), but the part that could immediately kill him isn't slamming into the ground.

As a professional, unless you are dealing with an armed opponent or multiple opponents, you should always try to hold the guy's head up as you take him down. This is especially true when you take him over backwards. It is a rare person who has the experience to instinctively tuck his chin into his chest when he falls over backwards. This will save you no end of shit. Not only are the courts less likely to charge you with murder or attempted murder, since it's not real likely that the guy is going to kick off without hitting his head, but it's harder to get a conviction for excessive force. Even the most nappy-headed granola-eating jury is less likely to believe that you were being a vicious authoritarian swine who brutally abused Poor Pitiful So-and-So if everyone saw you trying to protect his head when he went down.

Professionals

197

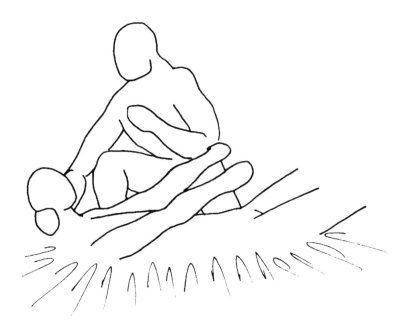

Figure 77. Catching his head.

Incidentally, if you had to physically move on someone, *make sure* that your report reads that you did everything possible to keep from hurting the guy. Maybe an expert will know what it was you were doing, but that isn't who is going to be sitting on the jury. Not only will this make it look better, but it will give your lawyer more ammo in your defense. If nothing else, you'll piss off the lawyer who's looking to sue by making his life more difficult, which is a worthwhile deed in any event. Go out and check into the necessary wording with your lawyer, but this kind of CYA is real handy to have up your sleeve.

Since it's sometimes almost fucking impossible to control someone without hurting him, the next best thing you can do is to not obviously hurt him while you're controlling him. It's what people *see* that is going to get your ass in trouble. Not only can one well-placed punch do more for you than five random blows with a tonfa, it can save you all sorts of shit down the line! If people only see you hit him once in a way they don't consider dangerous, they're not going to feel that you went ballistic and abused the guy, whereas those five tonfa strikes are going to look real bad regardless of how ineffective they really were. Face it, as professionals we cannot be seen to beat up on people.

When it comes to this kind of effectiveness, much of it comes from knowing human physiology, targets, and pressure points. Your one blow has to equal five of the average person's. For example, you can beat the shit out of a guy's rib cage and not stop him, whereas one good uppercut to his diaphragm will stop damn near anybody. Why? It's hard to keep on fighting when all the air is knocked out of you and that very thing that allows you to breathe is momentarily paralyzed.

This is in part what the attitude interrupters are about—doing one, maybe two moves that stun the dude long enough for you to get him down to the ground in order for you to control him. Somehow he's got to be struck hard enough that his attitude is derailed momentarily. While he's dwelling on the shock, you're busy either putting him into a controlled position or slapping the cuffs on him.

The advantage to all of this is that it's over quickly, the guy is put under control, and what everyone saw they won't consider unnecessarily brutal. I also gotta tell you that much of what you've learned in this book can and often is mistaken for the guy just losing his balance and falling down on his own. Oops, he rushed you and somehow in the scuffle he slipped and fell down (evil chuckle).

Let's say that you're in a situation where you have to not only control someone but move him along (like get his ass outside). Twirl the Way Back Machine to Figure 28—the backward takedown. From this position you can do one of two things: take him all the way down to the ground or take him just past his point of no return and then stop him from falling (Figure 78). This is a real awkward position for him and a real useful position for you, namely because people in this position can still walk but only in a direction you want them to . . . like toward the door.

Notice that the same hand that blew his center of gravity is now underneath him serving a dual purpose. It's supporting his torso weight and it's keeping him from levering himself back up.

You're not holding the guy in a chokehold while your arm is on his chest. This also serves a few purposes: it further serves to prevent him from regaining his balance, and it puts you in a perfect position to grab his head in case you have to drop him to drive home the point that he's made an unwise choice. Thirdly, his head, neck, and shoulders are resting against your torso, which is what really keeps him from suffering the effects of gravity, as that's where your really holding his weight up.

Incidentally, if the dude is really big or round, you may have to lift a knee up to help catch his falling weight so you can

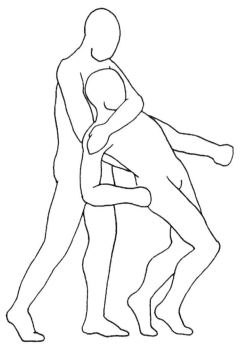

Figure 78.

get into position to support him. You catch his back across your thigh first to lessen the impact. Then you shift his weight to your torso. If you don't do this, his weight can knock you down if you're significantly smaller than him.

Once you've gotten someone into this position, if you step in any direction except backwards the guy is going to have to tiptoe around with you. If you step backward, odds are he's going to fall since the only thing keeping him up is you, and a backwards step removes that support. You can walk a guy out of a place this way with very little trouble or effort since he is supporting a good portion of his own weight. Remember to walk slow enough so his feet can keep pace in this difficult pose.

The real advantage of this hold is it allows you to drop someone who just isn't smart enough to realize exactly how bad a position he's in, but it puts the decision directly on him. Every time I've used it, I've immediately started a quick-talking monologue, reassuring the dude he won't be hurt if he cooperates. However if he tries to fight me I'll drop him. My voice is calm but authoritative. I talk fast so he can get the information he needs quickly to make an informed decision. This puts it in his lap. The only way he's going to get hurt is if he fights me.

If the dude is dumb enough, freaked-out enough, or drunk enough not to listen, then I have clearly stated for any witnesses that the only reason that I would take him down would be if he tries to attack again. Most of the time this works, but you still get those who are dumb enough to go for it.

In this situation you simply do a pivot/step to the side and let the dude fall (remembering to hold his head). As he's bouncing from the impact, flip him over onto his stomach and pin him down or wrist lock him. Let him think about having just slammed into the earth. If you're grabbing him didn't supply a big enough AI, then hitting the ground might just do the trick.

Professionals

For a moment I would like to address the bouncers out there. One thing that I really noticed from my last stint of bouncing was the number of them who really didn't understand the purpose of their job. By this I don't mean just the assholes who saw their job as an excuse to kick the shit out of someone. (They do exist out there. If you work with one, point it out to your boss, since it's his ass that the guy is going to get in the sling for sure, and maybe yours too.) I'm talking about the average run-of-the-mill bouncer. I want you to chew on the implications of what I am about to say. The purpose of a bouncer is *to protect the owner's interests!* Face it, you're a mercenary hired to protect something. What? The business. From what? From *all* threats, not just drunken fights!

Sure you cannot allow fights to go down. It's not only bad for business, but in most states if violence occurs you legally have to make a police report. If the owner or the manager doesn't, he's breaking the law. What happens if there's too many fights or too much violence in a place? The booze board and the cops shut it down. The reason you're there to keep fights from happening is to keep the bar open!

And this includes fights involving you! If you end up punching a dude out, odds are you're going to get fired if it's anything like an upscale place. You think the owner wants to get sued because you busted a drunk's jaw? Nope, you're history. That way the guy can claim that you were out of line and were fired because of it. That puts the misconduct (hence liability) on you.

Let's look at some of the other aspects of being a bouncer. What if the guy gets too intoxicated and gets in an accident? Why didn't you cut him off? Ooooh, bar faces liability. If the guy even enters your bar obviously sloshed and you let him in rather than refuse him entrance, the bar, and possibly you, may face fines. An underage kid breezes in without getting carded. The booze board walks in and starts checking IDs. Even if the dude is obviously over 21, if he has no identification to prove it, management is in some deep shit.

If the guy paws one of the girls and you don't throw him out, it's consensual sexual contact. Ooooo, that's prostitution, and you're now a participant in pandering. In comes the vice squad, down goes the bar. This is especially true in all nude and couch dance places. Are the girls dirty dancing while you're standing there watching? Indecent exposure. Not only does the girl get fined but so does the management. Are they touching the customers with certain parts of their bodies or grabbing on to rapidly enlarging tips? Ooohhh my.

Any and all of these can either get you fired or in deep shit, depending on how anal the state is. Yet when you ask most bouncers what their job is, they sort of shrug and say, "Keep fights from happening" or "Throw drunks out."

Sigh.

Perhaps the most depressing thing that I've noticed about bouncers is they very seldom know how to work as a team. Not only have I experienced this firsthand, but I've watched serious *Three Stooges* shit go down. Your life may depend on your partner not stepping on his dick at a critical moment, especially when you're dealing with a hard case instead of just your run-of-the-mill drunk.

Let me just point out a few of the more charming experiences that have come my way or I have seen as a bouncer.

An obnoxious drunk being dragged out into the parking lot and five bouncers beating him to the ground before they start kicking him.

The AssMan (of the topless bar I mentioned in the last chapter) and I walking up to three marines, one of whom had grabbed one of the girls a few minutes earlier. AssMan was in front of me and made first contact. As I drifted to the side, he simply declared, "Alright, you guys are out of here," grabbed their pitcher from the table, and then just turned and fucking walked away! I'm standing there facing three marines and he's heading toward the bar! They stand up and are thinking about tearing the place apart, starting with me. I start calmly talking and get them out the door. Later the AssMan gets upset when I and the manager jump down his throat. He didn't do anything wrong . . .

After having already gotten a young, steroid-pumped, obscenity-yelling drunk out the back door, with his friend trying to drag him away, having to body slam my partner against the wall to keep him from charging out into the parking lot and getting in a punch fest with the dude. Then I shoved him back inside and slammed the door so the drunk was facing a blank door and my "partner" had a short, furry, pissed-off guy between him and the door.

Seeing three bouncers chase a guy off the property into the street, catch him, drag him onto someone else's property, proceed to beat him until he fell, then start stomping him.

Standing there trying to get a drunk out and my fellow bouncer taking up position between the drunk and the door. Instead of herding him out the door, the drunk is now penned in the bar.

Watching a weightlifter walk up and wrap his arms around a guy and just pick him up and carry him to the door, without putting his head down to protect himself against possible headbutts.

Frantically running across the parking lot to stop a fellow bouncer who was totally ignoring what I had taught him about controlled takedowns. He had grabbed a guy in a chokehold, then hoisted him up by the throat to carry him off the property. To this day I can't believe he looked surprised when the dude passed out, slipped from his grip, and took a head dive into the asphalt. I'm standing there looking at him thinking to myself, "You just bought yourself a murder rap, asshole." (Fortunately, the dude was only knocked out.)

These are the sort of things that cause me to say that most bouncers really aren't professionals. They may be tough, they may be bad, but they are not professional about what they are doing. Here are a few tips on how to cover your ass legally and practically.

First of all, always remember that it's a job; it's nothing personal. Getting mad at an obnoxious drunk is really silly once you consider the source. Your job is to protect the owner's interest, not get your dick out of joint because some drunk asshole doesn't like the fact that you cut him off. If you don't react by getting angry, you remove much of what the drunk is going to use to justify going ballistic (it's called staying calm, firm, and polite).

You can't reason with a drunk. You can lie, bullshit, con, and trick one, but you can't reason with one. Another thing is you can always blame someone else. It's something drunks understand real well. Tell a drunk you can't serve him because it's the law, not your personal choice. If you served him you'd get in trouble. That makes you less of an asshole and more a victim of circumstance (just like him, at least according to him). I once sent a guy down to the state capitol of Arizona to complain about the unfairness of the law. It was just down the street, and he was drunk enough that walking into the capitol building and pitching a hissy fit seemed like a good idea. Sucker.

A subsidiary rule of this is that you don't have to be a tough guy all the time. You can lie like a rug if it just gets the dude out the door without you having to lay hands on him. Empathize with him, even if he's doing word salad (drunken babbling). Make up sisters and brothers to fit the story. Whatever. Just get him outside without flaming him off or having to dribble him. A screaming, belligerent drunk is bad for business, almost as bad as having to knock the shit out of him. If you can avoid such episodes by bullshitting, get your hip boots out!

Your goal is to get him outside the bar. Once he's outside, shut the door. Drunk or not, standing there screaming at a blank door really is not a satisfying experience. Most guys will wander away after a minute or two (naturally you check outside a few minutes later to make sure he has left and/or isn't trashing cars).

Never leave your partner facing someone alone! You never know when something is going to turn ugly. Ugly as in unexpected. If you think two bouncers at once will flash the guy over the edge, circle around from behind. Take up a post 5 to 10 feet away out of the dude's sight and just hang out until he is obviously leaving. Then trail along.

Go out and start looking up how to work as a team. Watch the true-life TV show "Cops" and take clues from how they move. Grab anybody you know who's ever worked with a partner and pump them for information on how to work with a partner when taking someone down. I've taken more elbows and accidental headbutts from partners than I have from the guys we were taking down! Especially remember that one of you talks while the other moves into position to drop the guy. You can save both of you loads of trouble this way.

Block every direction but the drunk's path to the door. Not only doesn't this make him feel trapped, hence less likely to fight, but it always leaves him the option of departing.

If you are a big old white boy, you had better listen to this one, because the effects can be deadly. Whenever you're dealing with a smaller opponent or someone from a different culture, keep in mind that he may have a weapon! Of all the things that I've seen that have sent me into shit fits, it's watching a big guy swagger up to a smaller opponent absolutely convinced that his size is going to take care of everything. The more experienced the smaller guy is, the more ugly it's going to be. Face it, a smaller, experienced guy has faced off bigger opponents before. You'd be flat-out stupid not to realize that the fact that he's still breathing implies that he's figured out something to even the odds. Then there's the politically incorrect but oh-so-accurate assumption that a guy from a different culture (or even different strata of the same culture) is carrying a weapon. With some groups you might as well just fill in the blank as "_____ = weapon."

Anytime you have to throw someone out real hard, be real careful about walking out the door at closing. In fact, it wouldn't hurt to trade off your post with someone who wasn't involved for about an hour or so. Make sure the guy knows what the dude looked like so he can keep an eye out for him. While it is possible that the guy will just walk in and open fire in general, most times he's going to come back looking for you in particular. Being in another position means that you will have a better chance of seeing him gunning for you.

Finally, be professional. As any cop can tell you, a professional attitude does wonders for keeping problems down. You've got nothing to prove; all you have is a job to do. And for God's sake, don't walk into a situation with the attitude that you can knock bullets out of the air with your dick unless you really want to put it to the test.

For the rest of you professionals, I recommend you go out and grab some of the old dogs who've lived through this and ask them what it was that they've been doing that kept their asses alive for so long. I always loved Sean Connery's quote from the movie *The Untouchables*, something along the lines of, "Any day that you're still alive at the end of your shift is a good day."

ENDNOTES

1. Normally the course for this step is planned out in childhood, before the testosterone hits. It's when the hormones get dumped in that the particular dysfunction is suddenly given *cajones*. (This is

another reason why I am so rabid against child abuse, as it's not only hurting the children and tribe, but it's making future predators.) However, the same change can occur with a severely traumatic experience (war for example) or a prolonged narrowing of focus (long-term brainwashing, for the lack of a better word). These two are much rarer than the first option.

2. Check out the movie *Jurassic Park* for a succinct summation of the situation. The science and evolutionary points it discusses are real.

3. The second-to-last straw for my leaving the directorship of the correctional center that I worked in was when my lady and I went into Pasadena and, in a beautiful brick courtyard with landscaped trellises and outdoor dining, I suddenly was struck with a realization that brought me up short. I stopped, looked around in confusion, and said in disbelief, "There are no felons here. All these people, and no one is a criminal or addict." I knew right then how bad the job was getting to me. I walked around in a euphoric daze for about 10 minutes just looking at people who had nothing to do with crime and violence. No criminals, no addicts, no cops, no lawyers, no judges, no parole officers, no prison bureaucrats.

4. The reason a clique is given power by society is because of the service it provides to that society. Once that service becomes secondary to the clique's continued power or internal needs, then it is no longer serving the real needs of society. At this moment it's real easy for it to become fascist/dictatorial.

5. That means nobody gets it entirely "their way," because if they did it would make it impossible for anyone else to function.

6. Not long ago at a class full of civilians, I was amazed to discover exactly how many men have *never* been in a fight in their lives. Not that such a thing is bad, but it gives them absolutely no real frame of reference regarding violence at all!

7. I personally only know of three occurrences where someone survived such a situation. Every one of them involved the guy wearing body armor and having an EMT/medic nearby.

8. The fact that head shots are often lethal probably has something to do with this assumption. I was reading somewhere that

something like 80 percent of all people who show up unconscious in hospital emergency rooms from traumatic head injuries die, and 50 percent of those who are conscious and can talk still croak. These are unconfirmed numbers, but you can begin to see why people would get bent out of shape about you going for the head.

Taking Away His Support

Afterword

> "*Professional soldiers are predictable, but the world is full of amateurs.*"
>
> —Murphy's Law of Combat #32

Being adept with tools is something that seems to run in my family. There must be something in my family's DNA that produces jacks-of-all-trades. But often that ability runs deeper than you'd think. There's something my grandfather once told me years ago that had a profound effect on my life: "You can figure anything out if you just look at it long enough."

Those simple words set off an avalanche inside my head. It eventually ended up with me being able to sit down and tell you things about physical violence and fighting in a way that, to the best of my knowledge, nobody else seems to do—that is, to get to the underlying fundamentals and tell you what they are and how they can manifest themselves. As a friend of mine says, I'm "a professional at stating the obvious."

Because honestly, that's all I'm doing here. Every time I sit down and write a book, I'm just telling you what is obvious to me—those underlying fundamentals that don't change no matter where you are or what's going on.

To tell you the truth, to me the manifestations are bullshit. "What technique do you use in this situation?" Man, the answer is never the same! I show the technique that I would use in that exact situation, but I know that that exact situation will never be recreated outside the academy! The reason is because every situation is different, and you must adapt to that, not try to adapt reality to your technique or wait until reality conveniently aligns itself to what you know! In this business, you bleed if you do that sort of shit.

With real violence, things shift, things change, Murphy's Law is out there. In other words, there are too many variables to either fixate on the details of the situation or only have one way of doing things. If you try to hang onto that mind-set (or are being taught by someone who has it), you're going to get hurt. But if you always remember the underlying fundamentals and tailor your actions to the details of a situation, you increase your chances of getting out of it in one piece. Remember, violence is not an academic exercise. The blood, the pain, and the damage are real. Because of this you can't afford to have misconceptions about it when you're facing it in real life.

That's where the comment, "You can figure anything out" comes in.

The key to that statement is patience. Most people want a fast, simple, convenient answer and get frustrated if they don't get one prepackaged. Walk around it and look at it from a few different perspectives, read a book or two about it, and then watch it operate. I cannot begin to tell you how powerful this tool really is. I am constantly asked, "Who taught you all of this?" Those same people are shocked when I tell them, "I figured it out." They either think I'm a total bullshit artist or some sort of messiah rather than a guy who just sat there, chewing on a stalk of grass, really watching the world, and then figuring out what it was that he saw.

I got news for you. Ninety percent of what you learn in the dojo came from some guy way back when who did the same thing. The problem is, although the technique remains today, not only has the original problem itself changed (how often have you been attacked by a sword-wielding samurai?), but the fact that it was really created by some poor shmuck who was trying to keep from getting his ass torn up has been forgotten! Maybe by the time the guy was 80 he was some sort of grand master, but when he figured it out he was just a regular guy like you and me! The only difference between him and everyone else is he somehow had stumbled across these fundamentals.

If he can do it, I can do it. If I can do it, you can do it. It's that simple. By knowing the fundamentals, you can do the same thing as I and Grand Master Whatshisnuts did—keep your ass alive in a live-fire situation! It's the same thing as understanding the basics of plumbing. Once you know the underlying way things work, you can identify and fix any problem you encounter, no matter how bad of a shit hole it is.

I've spent nearly 25 years of my life wrasslin' with violence, and one thing I've learned is that it's too serious of an issue for there to be academic bickering and egomaniacs teaching it to the poor guys who need it. It's not the instructor who's going to bleed for his fixating on the details, technique, or tradition; it's his students who will get hurt out there.

So you can go totally paranoid and learn 8,562,329 ways to fold/spindle/mutilate would-be attackers. You can fanatically dedicate yourself to a particular style (cheerleading dresses optional). You can learn a few simple techniques and hope you never end up in a situation where they won't work. Or you can learn the fundamental laws that everything stands on, spend some time playing around with how

Afterword

they manifest in different situations, keep them in mind, and then get on with your life.

I sort of like the last option. It's easy, it's flexible, you do some work on it for a while, and then carry on with other important stuff. How likely it is that you're going to get into the shit depends on how much time you spend working with the different manifestations. The more you know the fundamentals and have worked with their manifestations, the more the 8,562,329 techniques will just fall into line behind you. Pretty simple, but then again, "In any art there are few principles and many techniques" (Dale Carnegie, *How to Win Friends and Influence People*). Always remember the principles; don't get lost in the techniques.

Oh, by the way, these days it seems I'm never far from my computer. I can be reached through the Internet at:

AnimalMac@aol.com

Just don't expect a real coherent response before I've had my coffee.

Stages of Intoxication as Related to Violence

Alcohol is a depressant. It has a physiological effect on the human nervous system. This means the effects are physical before they are behavioral. While how someone will react to intoxication depends on their personality and experience with alcohol, the physical impairment to their system still exists.

The first parts of the brain that are affected by alcohol are the higher functions, i.e., logic, reasoning, learning, remembering, judgment, etc. These suppressed parts are the same that control moral reservations, behavioral modifiers, limits, and inhibitions. Putting it simply, the parts that keep a leash on a person's aggressive, violent, and sociopathic behavior are shut down. That leaves you with whatever is underneath the person's higher brain functions. If that part is violent, selfish, aggressive, or dysfunctional, you will have problems.

There are four stages of intoxication. I've included slang terminology as a guideline.

STAGE ONE:
Noticeable Alteration of Behavior (Buzzed)

As alcohol gradually begins to affect a person's physiology, he may begin to lose his inhibitions. A person may become noticeably emotional and demonstrate sudden and unexpected mood swings. Essentially, in this initial stage there is a general relaxation of behavior patterns. Many of these signs will appear immediately in inexperienced drinkers. Signs include uncharacteristic behavior; uncontrolled emotional displays; sudden, unexpected mood swings; becoming overtly friendly with strangers; brooding, detached, antisocial behavior; increased volume/boisterousness; acting in an annoying, irritating manner (pushy); loss of self-control; displays of immaturity; use of excessive profanity/crude or rude behavior; excessive touching; becoming animated, agitated, or entertaining.

STAGE TWO:
Temporary Disassociation (Drunk)

As an individual's blood alcohol concentration steadily increases, sensible action and rational thinking will diminish. Literally, a person can begin to phase into a psychotic or sociopathic state. With practiced drinkers, many of the symptoms described in Stage One will begin to appear in this stage either in lieu of or in tandem with Stage Two signs. Additional signs include diminished alertness; inability to make fine discriminations; increased rate of consumption (chug-a-lugging, drinking contests, etc.); moving onto straight shots of alcohol; short-term memory loss (not remembering what was just said to him); repeating a point he/she considers important; making irrational, unsubstantiated statements; aggressive, belligerent behavior; displays of bravado; confrontational and argumentative behavior.

STAGE THREE:
Impairment to Normal Brain Function (Bombed)

Alcohol will not only slow down brain activity, it will impair normal brain functions. As blood alcohol concentration increases, activities that normally require no conscious thought, such as lighting cigarettes, speaking clearly, or walking, gradually become more difficult. Signs of this stage include difficulty lighting cigarettes (lighting the wrong end, two cigarettes at once); glassy and unfocused eyes, dilated pupils; loss of eye contact, reduced visual acuity; loss of concentration and sequence of thought (digressing or trailing off and not finishing sentences); altered speech patterns (talkativeness, exaggerated or deliberate speech); drowsiness, drooping eyelids, nodding off; reactive, confrontational behavior, temper tantrums.

STAGE FOUR:
Loss of Dexterity and Muscle Control
(Wasted, Fucked Up, Polluted)

As the alcohol begins to affect the central nervous system, a person's coordination will steadily deteriorate to a point where simple tasks become impossible. Hand/eye coordination, dexterity, balance, and motor functions are severely impaired. The ability to have an erection is also suppressed. This is the final stage before passing out. Unlike other levels where a certain amount of competence remains, this level of impairment makes him basically incompetent at violence. Nonetheless, the potential for belligerence still remains, although much of what is said is "word salad" and incomprehensible to an outsider.

With all of these stages it is important to realize that the effects of alcohol intensify up to 25 percent in the hour following the last drink. A person can quit drinking and still slip into the next stage of intoxication. When it comes to the effects of alcohol on a person, a good way of looking at it is to imagine layers of self-control being peeled away with every drink. Depending on what is underneath determines what will come to the surface when enough layers are removed. If the person is violent or selfish, each stage of intoxication increases the likelihood of attack/violence as the barriers are removed.

The two most common types of violence to occur under the influence of alcohol are tantrum and frenzy, although the possibility of the other two (fear and criminal) also exist (more on common types of violence in appendices C and D). The tantrum is especially applicable for drunk/nondrunk confrontations, as alcohol is often used as an excuse for violence rather than being the cause. In situations like this, the person has a pre-existing anger when he started drinking, and the alcohol is used to counter the inhibitors against violence. In other words, he was in a bad mood when he started drinking and he's looking for trouble. The person wants the release of violence and is drinking for that purpose. The most extreme case of this is an abuser who drinks for the sole reason of an excuse for beating his wife or children. It is a well-known dynamic for young males, upon realizing that they are not going to find a sexual partner that evening, to rechannel that energy into conflict. Even the person who drinks "to blow off steam" is following this same pattern but to varying degrees. Often at the first sign of resistance to their actions, these people proceed to spin on the path of tantrum violence.

The frenzy type of violence is most common among two or more drinkers. Much of this is based on the fact that alcohol removes the higher functions and leaves emotions raw. Something occurs, such as a comment by another person, that delivers an emotional impact. This can act as a provocation to start the escalation. Without the higher functions to set boundaries on emotional responses, the situation can escalate into violence. This is often seen in the drunken quarrel, where two impaired people flailing about with verbal violence become caught up in an escalating spiral into a frenzy state. At this point neither person perceives boundaries or limits and is operating purely on an emotional level.

Unless the person is severely antisocial to begin with, the chances of an attack occurring during the first stage of intoxication are slim (although it is possible). Commonly, the most dangerous periods are Stages Two and Three, where the person has inhibited judgment but remains physically able to commit an attack. Again, fourth stage violence will not be at any level of competence.

Effects of Alcohol on Higher Brain Functions

U nder normal circumstances, the higher brain functions serve to control baser instincts and aggressive behavior. If one were to do a percentage breakdown, it might look something like the wheel below. This is the basis for most people's normal behavior.

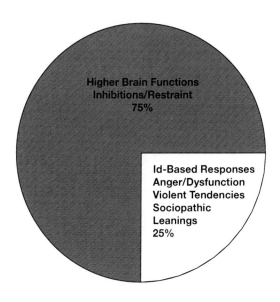

Higher Brain Functions
Inhibitions/Restraint
75%

Id-Based Responses
Anger/Dysfunction
Violent Tendencies
Sociopathic
Leanings
25%

However alcohol causes a physiological suppression of the higher brain functions. This leaves whatever is underneath those functions dangerously close to the surface.

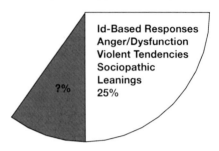

TEMPORARILY OUT OF SERVICE

Id-Based Responses
Anger/Dysfunction
Violent Tendencies
Sociopathic
Leanings
25%

?%

How much of the higher functions remain depends on 1) the amount and type of alcohol consumed, 2) how well in place the higher functions were to begin with, and 3) the attitude of the person before intoxication. While this works as a good rule of thumb, realize that even the best-behaved person can turn hostile when confronted with disappointment or frustration of his desires while intoxicated.

Four Types of Violence

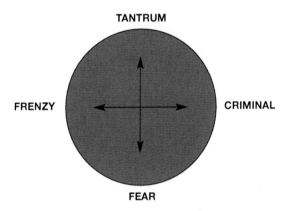

FEAR: Violence based in the person feeling threatened.

FRENZY: Violence based in the person not perceiving external limits or boundaries (self-feeding internal images overriding external information; "flip out/spin out").

TANTRUM: Violence based on escalating tantrum behavior (pre-existing and/or chronic anger being directed outward).

CRIMINAL: Violence used as coercion (violence for profit, whether monetary or perceived, i.e., power or position).

Arrows indicate the most likely way that violence patterns will shift from one type to another.

The Four Types of Violence and Their Counters

There are four basic mental states that lead to violence. These are referred to as "types of violence" or "patterns." As poisons have antidotes that counteract their effects, each type of violence has a "response" that is most likely to de-escalate the situation and prevent it from becoming physical.

The four types of violence are fear, frenzy, tantrum, and criminal. Failing to approach a certain type with the appropriate response will, instead of stopping it, actually feed the process and result in violence.[1] It is critical for the person to correctly identify the type of situation that he/she is facing.

FEAR

Fear-based violence is based in the person's perception that he is being threatened (by a person, group, or situation). Whether this reaction is based in neurosis, chemicals, or actual stimuli, the person will panic and attempt to fight his way free. For example, it is extremely common for a single, smaller person to become unnerved when surrounded by a group of large individuals. He doesn't see that his reactions have any bearing on the situation (i.e., they won't attack if he calms down); he instead only perceives the other's "aggression" and reacts accordingly. In this situation, a person in the fear mental state will "counterattack" despite any and all odds.

Response: The technique of dealing with a fear state is found in mimicry. It's convincing him that you are just as scared as he is and therefore no threat. When approaching a person in a fear state, adopt a hunched over, nonthreatening position. The voice should reflect fear state—use a high-pitched, breathy voice with a cadence similar to the scared person's. Empty hands are held in front in clear view and make petting (calming) gestures. You have to "go out after him" and bring that person back from fear. Once the person is calmed down, the situation can be resolved. Any display of aggression or dictatorial behavior will set the person off, as it reinforces the fear the person is feeling.

FRENZY

A person in a frenzy state does not perceive limits or balances. The brakes have been taken off the situation and it is spinning out of control. Basically, the person is looking at the situation from an extreme point of view and is disregarding anything that would contradict this perspective, while simultaneously fixating on things that will perpetuate it. All he can see is a huge, looming, emotional image in his mind's eye. This internal image is what serves as the basis for his actions, not what is actually occurring around him. This is an inwardly based problem, where the person that you are dealing with is not really "here" in the present. He is "off deep" inside his own mind or emotions. The more energy and thought that the person pours into this mental process, the more extreme the situation will become.

Now it often does occur that the person is reacting to a real external situation; however, he takes it and then runs with it. This sort of situation can happen by the person legitimately undergoing more than he/she can bear and exploding. However, more often it is a case of a person who encounters a limit/boundary and then fixates on why he "must" get around it. He "has" to do something a certain way, and he is willing to commit violence to do so. A third, and the most common variation is a situation between two people that has escalated out of control (usually influenced by alcohol and/or drugs). This is a drunken quarrel that has gotten out of hand. It is up to an intervening third party to reestablish boundaries.

Response: The way to handle this type of situation is to provide stimuli that overrides the person's internal process. It snaps him back into reality by forcing him outside of his own head. This is classic pattern interruption, as it derails his train of thought and forces him to focus on something else other than himself. An authoritarian demeanor and loud, commanding voice are used. Personal space invasion, "baton gestures" with the hand, and an immediate removal of options is needed to snap the person outside of his own head and back into reality.

Limiting the person's options is critical. Via a specific command, the person is given no option except to respond or face the consequences. If compliance is not gained immediately, the command is given in stronger terms until compliance is gained. If by the third time an order is given the person fails to comply, physical action is applied to put him into the ordered state. The original order is restressed during this process. For example, if you tell someone to sit on the curb and he refuses, you only tell him three times. The next thing that person knows is he is slammed into a sitting position. At this point, instead of more physical action, immediately get in his face and again repeat the order, thereby also stressing your authority over him in the here and now. Restating the order while the person is in shock of being physically manhandled is important, as it immediately establishes a connection between noncompliance and punishment. It also establishes that compliance means he will not be punished more.

The Four Types of Violence and Their Counters

TANTRUM

This is the most confusing of all types of violence and the most difficult to handle for anyone not professionally trained. It is based in internalized anger, which is outwardly directed. Literally, it is an explosion looking for an excuse to happen.

This type of violence often seems to skip steps of the normal process of escalation, leaving the victim bewildered by both the speed and the unexpected intensity of the process. Unlike normal anger, where a person builds up to a violent state, a tantrum type is already to that point and is looking for an excuse to explode or is trying to creating one. While it is common for this behavior to be directed toward weaker victims (i.e., abuse or bullying), it can as often be directed at someone who is competent in the area of physical conflict. In both cases, alcohol is often involved.

In the case of weaker victims, tantrum behavior commonly manifests as a "demanding" process, where the person is demanding some form of attention/behavior/article/money from the victim. The bullying demands escalate in degree and become more intense and unrealistic until they can no longer be met. (For example, "Gimme a cigarette. Gimme a CAMEL! GIMME A CAMEL FILTER!") It is at this time that the violence occurs.

Another type of tantrum can occur where the person is literally looking for a fight. He engages in conduct that he knows will draw attention from either a bystander or an authority figure. Once a boundary is established, he proceeds to direct his anger at the person who "interfered" with him. This is the most common type of violence in bars between a drunk and bouncer. The best way to recognize a tantrum situation is the rising sense of confusion that you get when confronted with the person's unreasonable demands or anger.

Response: The person in a tantrum state is basically demanding negative attention and is trying to escalate the situation to the point where he can explode. He's actively looking for an excuse to attack someone! This explosion acts as a release for his surplus anger. This is why this type of violence is so confusing to the average person, as it appears to be a no-win situation. Compliance or refusal both will result in violence.

The way to handle this situation effectively is a two-part process. One is to refuse to fuel the fire while stopping the behavior. This is done by withdrawing emotional attention or feedback. The person in this state will take any emotional response on your part and use it as an excuse to escalate the situation. You must establish that not only will the demands not be met, but this behavior will not be tolerated. Furthermore, until a different approach is used, emotional feedback will be withdrawn from the tantrum thrower. At best you adopt a professionally polite and unattached manner and at worst a demeanor that would give a "Terminator" frostbite. In the latter, the eyes are "dead" and the voice is flat and atonal with no emotional attachment to the inflection. The body is held in a neutral, ready pose. A direct and repeated order is given that is the equivalent of "go sit in the corner until you can behave." Until that person chooses to alter his behavior, there is no feedback given to him on an emotional level.

The second part to this process is the willingness to immediately match whatever level of violence the tantrum thrower might initiate. Since the threat of violence is the tantrum thrower's ace in the hole, calm competence is exuded to offset the implied threat. No overt threat is made, but a quiet readiness for action is projected. It should be noted that tantrum throwers often "feint" with abortive attacks or intimidating gestures. If the person facing the tantrum reacts to these gestures in fear and/or an overly defensive manner, the situation will become unmanageable, as the tantrum thrower will interpret it as both an emotional reaction and a sign of fear. In these situations, the person facing the feint must either not react at all or immediately overwhelm the tantrum thrower. This is not a "fight," as you must be ready, willing, and able to slam the tantrum thrower into a wall and contain him.

CRIMINAL

Criminal violence is basically coercion. The victim is told that they have only two choices: surrender something or face the consequences. "Do what I want or I will hurt you." Any time a person is placed in a situation where refusing to surrender to another's wishes will result in physical injury, that situation can be defined as criminal violence.

Response: The response to criminal violence is incredibly easy. It is to renegotiate the contract. Remove the binary option of compliance or victimization and replace it with the following: "Any attempt to force this ultimatum will be met with resistance equal or greater than the attack." For example, "If you try to attack me, I will hurt you."[2] I cover this topic in great detail in my video *Safe in the Street*.

ENDNOTES

1. In the area of obvious authority, i.e., police or hospital orderly, if violence is not the end result, it will result in more difficulty containing the situation.

2. Thanks to Richard Dobson for the core concepts of this system.

Four Quads/Quarters and Windows

The human body can be divided into four quarters from the center of gravity (CG). Each quadrant is susceptible to attack. When an attack occurs, generally it only threatens one particular quadrant. In certain cases this can be increased to two. Safety comes by removing the threatened quadrant from the line of attack.

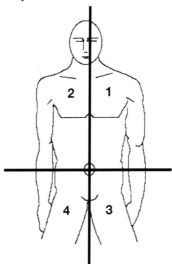

In a related issue, by the fact that we only have two hands, a person can only protect two quadrants at a time. This means that the person will, no matter what his hand placement, leave two other quadrants exposed, thereby creating "windows" in his defense. It is through these holes or windows that you target your attack.

You can make an immediate assessment of a person's fighting ability (and threat level) by considering what he is exposing behind these windows. A person who automatically covers these windows and moves his body away from his open windows is not someone you want to engage in an extended conflict with.

Learn to look for the windows that someone leaves open. An instinctive and immediate understanding of this principle will show you where to focus your attacks.

Certain sports training will often cause a person to expose sections of the quadrants in addition to the normal

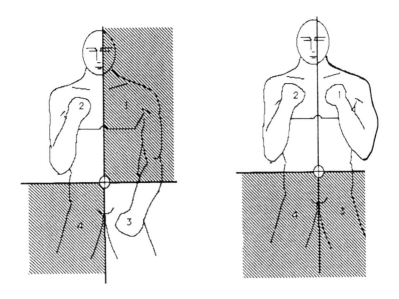

two. This is because certain moves are not allowed in sports contests. This sort of person is usually susceptible to kicks and attacks to his legs. However care should be taken, as some skilled fighters will intentionally leave gaps in their defenses as traps.

Two Feet and Stance Integrity

TWO FEET AND STANCE INTEGRITY

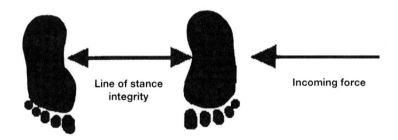

Line of stance integrity

Incoming force

Unless you're fighting a mutant, your opponent will only have two feet. No matter what stance he assumes, there is an inherent weakness in it. Any two points can have a line drawn between them. This line between two feet is the "line of stance integrity." There is stability against any incoming force along this line (or in close relationship to it). The wider the distance between these two points, the more a person will be able to resist an incoming force. In this case, the force necessary to move the person must be significantly increased to overcome the

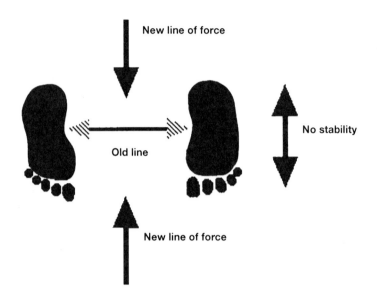

New line of force

Old line

No stability

New line of force

stance integrity. Simply stated, "That is too much like work." However, a force coming in perpendicular (90 degrees) to the line of stance integrity has no such limitations to overcome.

Without the line of stance integrity to stabilize the person against the incoming force, the only thing keeping the person standing would be his ability to redeploy his feet. If the force is delivered sufficiently fast enough, this is not likely. No matter what size a person is or how well he is "trained," this weakness exists and can be exploited by you.

Anything up to 45 degrees in either direction (totaling a 90-degree vector) off the person's stance integrity is likely to resist any force coming in from that area. This works to either side. Of the total 360 degrees, 180 of those are going to be able to resist force. The remaining two are the effective angles of attack.

By drawing an X where the person is standing, you can figure out which direction his stance integrity is. Once that

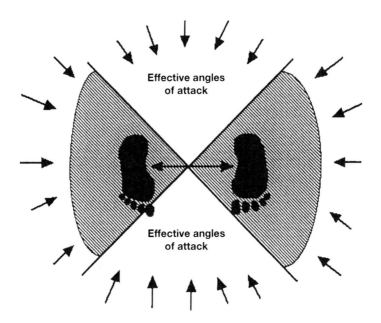

Effective angles of attack

Effective angles of attack

is established, then you can attack through the remaining two sectors.

Being able to immediately and instinctively recognize a person's line of stance integrity will give you the ability to instantly end a conflict by knocking your opponent off his feet. Once he's down, you can gain control with locking techniques or break off the engagement and flee.

Murphy's Laws of Combat

1. You are not a superman.
2. If it's stupid but works, it isn't stupid.
3. Don't look conspicuous—it draws fire.
4. When in doubt, empty your magazine.
5. Never share a foxhole with anyone braver than you are.
6. Never forget that your weapon was made by the lowest bidder.
7. If your attack is going really well, it's an ambush.
8. No plan survives the first contact intact.
9. All five-second grenade fuses will burn down in three.
10. Try to look unimportant because the bad guys may be low on ammo.
11. If you are forward of your position, the artillery will fall short.
12. The enemy diversion you are ignoring is the main attack.
13. The important things are always simple.
14. The simplest things are always hard.
15. The easy way is always mined.
16. If you are short of everything except enemy, you are in combat.

17. When you have secured an area, don't forget to tell the enemy.
18. Incoming fire has the right of way.
19. Friendly fire—isn't.
20. If the enemy is in range, SO ARE YOU!
21. Beer math is 2 beers x 37 men = 49 cases.
22. No combat-ready unit has ever passed inspection.
23. Body count math is 2 dead guerrillas + 1 portable + 2 pigs = 37 enemy killed in action.
24. Things that must be together to work usually can't be shipped together.
25. Radios will fail as soon as you desperately need fire support.
26. Anything you do can get you shot, including doing nothing.
27. Tracers work both ways.
28. The only thing more accurate than incoming enemy fire is incoming friendly fire.
29. Make it tough for the enemy to get in and you can't get out.
30. If you take more than your fair share of objectives you'll have more than your fair share of objectives to take.
31. When both sides are convinced that they are about to lose, they're both right.
32. Professional soldiers are predictable, but the world is full of amateurs.
33. Murphy was a grunt.

Thank you, Mr. Murphy, whoever you are. You said it all.

Applied Self-Defense Laws and Their Reasons

1. **The objective is to live long enough to lie to your grandkids.**
   This is long-term survival, not fighting. Take no unnecessary punishment.

2. **When two tigers fight, one dies, the other is wounded.**
   Win or lose, you're gonna get hurt. Avoid when possible; if you can't, win. It hurts less.

3. **The quicker it ends, the less likely you are to get hurt.**
   This ain't a game. Get him down with you in control and/or you gone ASAP.

4. **When you're up to your ass in alligators . . .**
   Neutralize the threat first, then think about counterattacking.

5. **Be a mongoose, not a bull.**
   Fight and flight in accord. Which one is happening is subject to change without notice.

6. **In the end, victory is won by those who made the fewest mistakes.**
    Win not by having more power but by having it more together than your attacker.

7. **Your best weapon is your mind.**
    Mental flexibility arms you better than them. Of course, mental flexibility and a .45 . . .

8. **Everything's got its limits, weaknesses, and counters.**
    Know them, and when you encounter one, stop doing whatever it is you're doing.

9. **You're not an ape, use a tool.**
    Anything can be used as a weapon. This isn't time for Marquis of Queensberry rules.

10. **What isn't there is just as important as what is there.**
    Strike through his weaknesses, don't contest his strengths. Expect him to do likewise.

11. **When the enemy is in range, SO ARE YOU!**
    Anyone can be counterattacked. Plan for it and all your surprises will be pleasant.

12. **Murphy's Law works in spades in this biz.**
    Keep it as simple as possible 'cause the other guy ain't on your side.

13. **Hit through his blind spot, from behind, and at any weaknesses.**
    Blindside him whenever you can. Remember, this isn't fighting, it's surviving.

14. **It ain't over till it's over.**
    It doesn't end with a body on the floor. Plan for that before you move.

15. **Righteousness won't help you in a fight.**
    Once violence starts, right or wrong doesn't matter, surviving does.

16. **Professionals are predictable, but the world is full of amateurs.**
    Along with the competent, expect the unexpected, crazed, and stupid.

17. **FUCK THE ART, GET THE JOB DONE!**
    'Nuff said.

Comments Regarding the Trigger

Some people have asked me what standards they should use to activate a trigger. Well, mine is pretty simple. My trigger goes off whenever someone physically attacks me with the intent to hurt me. You can stand there and scream obscenities in my face all day long and I won't get too bent. You can huff and puff all you want and I still won't move. There are even some people out there who I don't really consider a physical threat even when they move on me. I've sucked up a blow or two from these folks and didn't go ballistic on them, or I just did what I had to do to contain them. This is because I have two different triggers: one professional and one personal. However, make a dedicated attack on me and you'll meet the second one. I'll slam your face into the ground at 90+ mph in under 3 seconds.

While each type of violence—fear, frenzy, tantrum, and criminal—has its own flavor, build up, and warning signs, there is a particular habit common to tantrum types you should know about. The odds of meeting this kind of behavior go up astronomically if you are in a profession that brings you into confrontation with assholes. *It is real common that they will make a feint at you!* What they do is some sort of fast action that looks like an attack, but then they abort before having to commit. Quite literally, they do every part of an attack except throw the punch. They're angry, they lunge, they jerk their shoulders, they may even lift their hands, but they stop before they actually have to throw the punch. If this reminds you of something you underwent in high school, it's because it is a refinement of the same stupid shit action. However now it has more dangerous overtones.

First off, know it's a game. It's a conscious attempt at setting you up. *It is him testing to see if he's scaring you!*

How you react will determine how the situation will turn out. React correctly and he'll back off; react wrong and it becomes violent. In this case, the wrong reaction qualifies as anything that convinces him that you are scared of mixing it up. In other words, any purely defensive action is the wrong one.

Oddly, what qualifies as "right" in this situation doesn't really look it until you recognize a few other mitigating circumstances. If you react by jumping or flinching to his fake attack, then you're scared of him and he's got the upper hand, at least in his mind, which unfortunately determines if he attacks or not. Why? He did a pseudoattack and all you did was go defensive. That means you ain't got the balls to take it all the way. This is a gross simplification, but it is a good rule of thumb of what is going on inside his head if you just drop into a defensive stance.

Of course if you react by stomping the shit out of him, he claims that you started it, and that's what most people will remember.

The most common feint is the shoulder drop, where the guy drops his shoulder as if he's about to punch. This may or may not be combined with the raising of the fist, depending on how experienced the dude is (read: obvious). There you are, confronting this guy who's snorting and hollering, and suddenly in the middle of it all it looks like he's just crossed the line and is coming at you. However, unless a witness is well trained to recognize such nuances, to their way of seeing it you two were arguing and all of a sudden you went ballistic on the dude. Now, which of the 5,000 jerks and twitches that occurred during your confrontation was the one you claim justified your attack?

Begin to see the trap yet? Even if the dude gets his ass kicked, he still gets the satisfaction of getting your ass in trouble for attacking him!

Your best bet for handling this sort of shit is to "obviously" ignore it, while on a deeper level send messages to the dude that he's about to have his liver ripped out through his throat if he doesn't cut that shit out. Some of the tricks I've used are just standing there in my ready pose, calmly taking my sunglasses out of my pocket and tossing them into a nearby planter, turning my baseball hat backwards, and handing my radio to someone else.

You can also have no end of fun calling the guy's game with witty (and quiet) comments like, "You sure about that?" "Feeling lucky, sport?" and, of course, "Go for it." None of these can be taken as you doing anything to provoke an attack. Legal responsibility for the attack still resides with him, especially if you said it low enough and nobody else heard. One of these comments quietly snarled in response to his feint lets him know in no uncertain terms that you know exactly what he's up to and that he ain't going to get away with it. It also implies both viciousness and cunning on your part. Not a safe thing to mess with.

Of course, all of these work much better when combined with the murderous glare. Nothing else moves, but suddenly laughing boy is looking into the eyes of a very large, very pissed predator. My murderous glare has been described as a "werewolf looking at lunch." When the guy feints, my only reaction is to look him straight in the eyes with a gaze that says he's just moved into the second trigger territory for pulling that shit and the moment he moves for real, all bets are off. Once it turns physical, I will drink his blood, and I'll enjoy it. Not because he's a threat, but because he's pissed me off by pulling that shit.[1]

By not being suckered into his fake, you don't give him the actions he's going to use to justify his behavior. Believe it or not, that's important to the human psyche. Even the most twisted, messed-up person is running a game of justification inside his head. He was justified in doing this because . . ., or he had to because . . . well, he was upset at the time, etc., etc. The list is endless, and you'll grow old and die before people run out of excuses and justifications for their bad behavior.

There is a predictable and underlying process to this kind of reasoning, which you can use to your advantage. In any event, one of the best ways to de-escalate a situation is to not give the guy the parts he needs to complete his justification process. In this case, by not supplying him, you can prevent it from becoming violent.

Bullies feel safe behaving this way because they know that other people don't normally play outside the rules. Most bullies know where the line is, and they intentionally push it to see if they can get away with it.

Decide beforehand which trigger you need to handle any situation.[2] However if the dude starts up with this feint shit, either drop his ass in a controlled takedown right then and there or ignore it (NOT!). However, let him know that you've just moved the trigger level up one notch because he's pushing it. Since the most effective form of this is to broadcast it nonverbally, what can he say? "He looked at me with death in his eye?" Man, any lawyer will make mincemeat out of that statement alone. Nobody else needs to know that you're going to lay in some serious punishment on the dude for running this game on you, just you and him, and it's all in the look.

ENDNOTES

1. This is called "putting a price tag on bad behavior." It also works if you tell a bully that you're in a good mood and don't want to fight, but if he insists on pushing it, you're going to hurt him extra special for fucking up your good mood. I have kept my word to assholes who've kept it up with that special added set of cracked ribs, busted hand/arm, or crushed knee after it's all over. It isn't a fight anymore. The last shot is the promised punishment.

2. While I hope you will wire in both kinds of triggers, getting them both does take some time and experience. If you only go for one, I'd recommend the first one (not to kill but to end and contain). Remember, the kid you're supposed to send through school is yours, not your lawyer's.